Fundamentals of Machine Learning and Deep Learning in Medicine

Reza Borhani • Soheila Borhani •
Aggelos K. Katsaggelos

Fundamentals of Machine Learning and Deep Learning in Medicine

Springer

Reza Borhani
Electrical and Computer Engineering
Northwestern University
Evanston, IL, USA

Soheila Borhani
Biomedical Informatics
University of Texas Health Science Center
Houston, TX, USA

Aggelos K. Katsaggelos
Electrical and Computer Engineering
Northwestern University
Evanston, IL, USA

ISBN 978-3-031-19501-3 ISBN 978-3-031-19502-0 (eBook)
https://doi.org/10.1007/978-3-031-19502-0

This Springer imprint is published by the registered company Springer Nature Switzerland AG
The registered company address is: Gewerbestrasse 11, 6330 Cham, Switzerland

To our families:

Maryam and Ali
Ειρηνη, Ζωη, Σοφια and Adam

Preface

Not long ago, machine learning and deep learning were esoteric subjects known only to a select few at computer science and statistics departments. Today, however, these technologies have made their way into every corner of the academic universe, including medicine. From automatic segmentation of medical imaging data, to diagnosing medical conditions and disorders, to predicting clinical outcomes, to recruiting patients for clinical trials, machine learning and deep learning models have produced results that rival, and in some cases exceed, human performance. These groundbreaking successes have garnered the attention of healthcare stakeholders in academia and industry, with many anticipating and advocating for an overhaul of current educational curricula in order to prepare students for the transition of medicine from the "information age" to the "age of AI."

As medical and health-related programs begin to incorporate machine learning and deep learning into their curricula, a salient question arises about the extent to which these subjects should be taught, given that researchers and practitioners in these fields can, and often do, use various forms of technology without full knowledge of their inner-workings. For instance, a diagnostician need not necessarily be familiar with how magnetic fields are generated inside a scanner machine in order to interpret an MRI accurately. Similarly, surgeons can learn to operate robotic surgical systems effectively without ever knowing how to build, fix, or maintain one. We believe the same cannot be said about the use of artificial intelligence in medicine. For example, oncologists cannot be the mere end-users of a machine learning model which recommends the best course of treatment for a given cancer patient. They need to understand how these models work and, ideally, play an active role in developing them. Otherwise, one of two scenarios is bound to occur: either physicians will uncritically accept the model recommendations (which is a dangerous form of automation bias), or they will learn to distrust and ignore such recommendations to the detriment of their patients who could benefit from the "wisdom" of data-driven models trained on millions upon millions of examples.

Thanks to the immense popularity of machine learning and deep learning, the market abounds with textbooks written on these subjects. However, having generally been written *by* mathematicians and engineers *for* mathematicians and engineers, these texts are not geared toward the specific educational needs of medical students, researchers, and practitioners. Put differently, they are written in a "language" which is not accessible to the average scholar in medicine who typically lacks a graduate-level background in mathematics and computer science. Nearly six decades ago, the pioneering British medical scientist Sir Harold Percival Himsworth addressed this very challenge in his opening statement to the 1964 Conference on Mathematics and Computer Science in Biology and Medicine: "Medical biologists, mathematicians, physicists and computologists may have more of their outlook in common than we suspect. But they do speak different dialects and they do have different points of view. This is no new problem for a multidisciplinary subject like medical research. If it is to be solved and the evident necessity for co-operation realized, one thing is essential: we must learn each other's language."

The book before you is an attempt to realize this vision by providing an accessible introduction to the fundamentals of machine learning and deep learning in medicine. To serve an audience of medical researchers and professionals, we have presented throughout the book a curated selection of machine learning applications from medicine and adjacent fields. Additionally, we have prioritized intuitive descriptions over abstract mathematical formalisms in order to remove the veil of unnecessary complexity that often surrounds machine learning and deep learning concepts. A reader who has taken at least one introductory mathematics course at the undergraduate level (e.g., biostatistics or calculus) will be well-equipped to use this book without needing any additional prerequisites. This makes our introductory text appropriate for use by readers from a wide array of medical backgrounds who are not necessarily initiated in advanced mathematics but yearn for a better understanding of how these disruptive technologies can shape the future of medicine.

Evanston, IL, USA — Reza Borhani
Houston, TX, USA — Soheila Borhani
Evanston, IL, USA — Aggelos K. Katsaggelos

Contents

Chapter 1
Introduction

Throughout history, humans have always sought to better understand the natural phenomena that directly impacted their lives. Precipitation is one example. For eons, the ability to predict rainfall was the holy grail for our ancestors whose livelihoods were continuously under threat by prolonged droughts and major floods. Oblivious to the principles of hydrology and out of desperation, some resorted to human sacrifice[1] in the hope of pleasing the gods and saving their crops. The enlightenment brought about a drastic change in the way we think about the phenomena of interest to us, replacing religious and philosophical dogmas with the tools of scientific reasoning and experimentation. For instance, it was through careful and repeated experimentation that Galileo discovered the parabolic nature of projectile motion, as described in his book: "Dialogues concerning two new sciences" [1]. Galileo's discovery refuted the long-lasting Aristotelian theory of linear motion and paved the way for precise calculation of the trajectory of cannonballs as the most advanced weaponry of his time (see Fig. 1.1). Decades later, Isaac Newton formalized Galileo's observations through a set of differential equations that fully describe the behavior of virtually all moving objects around us, cannonballs included.

At the dawn of the third decade of the third millennium, we no longer pray to gods for rain, nor do we keep our fingers crossed during wartime for artillery shells to hit their intended targets. As a civilization, we are now capable of creating artificial rain (via cloud seeding) and launching intercontinental ballistic missiles with pinpoint accuracy. The unsolved problems of today are much more complex by comparison, an example of which are human maladies such as cancers and auto-immune disorders that, despite our best efforts, continue to claim the lives of millions every year. To compare the complexity of these modern problems with

[1] The Aztecs would sacrifice their young children before *Tlaloc*, the god of water and earthly fertility. Mayans believed that the rain god *Chaac* would strike the clouds with his lightning axe to cause thunder and rain.

R. Borhani et al., *Fundamentals of Machine Learning and Deep Learning in Medicine*, https://doi.org/10.1007/978-3-031-19502-0_1

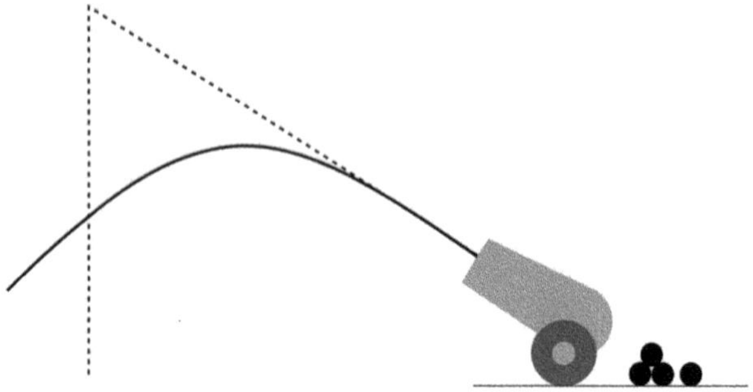

Fig. 1.1 The path taken by projectiles according to Aristotle (dashed lines) and Galileo (solid parabola)

those of the past, consider, as an example, the second law of motion in Newtonian mechanics. This well-known law, expressed commonly as $\mathbf{F} = m\,\mathbf{a}$, states that the acceleration **a** of any moving object is influenced by *two factors* only: the object's mass m and the net force **F** exerted on it. Additionally, the relationship between acceleration and force happens to be *linear*, which is the easiest to model mathematically. Furthermore, this simple linear relationship is *universal* meaning that it applies similarly to all moving objects and at all times, regardless of their location, speed, and other physical attributes.

In contrast, diseases are not single-factor or bi-factor phenomena. A mathematical model of cancer (if one is ever to be discovered) would likely include tens of thousands of genetic and environmental variables. In addition, these variables may not necessarily interact in a conveniently linear fashion, making their mathematical modeling immensely more difficult. Finally, there is no universality with human diseases as they do not always manifest the same across all afflicted individuals. As a result of this inherent variance and complexity, traditional mathematical machinery and deductive reasoning tools employed to solve many classical chemistry and physics problems in the centuries past cannot adequately address the complex biology problems of the twenty-first century.[2]

Luckily for us, we have at our disposal today an extremely valuable commodity that we can utilize when modeling complex phenomena: *data*. Unlike our forefathers who did not possess the technology to generate and store large quantities of data, we live in a world awash in it. Currently, more than two zettabytes (i.e., 2×10^{21} bytes) of medical data are generated annually across the globe in the form of electronic health records, high-resolution medical images, bio-signals, genome sequencing data, and more. These massive amounts of data are easily accessible through large distributed networks of interconnected servers dubbed "the cloud."

[2] The development of the atomic model and the periodic table of elements revolutionized chemistry in the nineteenth century. In the twentieth century, physics underwent a paradigm shift with the advent of quantum mechanics. Many believe that the complete mapping of the human genome coupled with the ongoing information technology revolution promises similar leaps of progress for biology in the twenty-first century.

This over-abundance of data has reshaped many scientific disciplines including artificial intelligence (AI). One of the first applications of AI in medicine was a chat-bot named ELIZA [2] created by Joseph Weizenbaum at the Massachusetts Institute of Technology in 1964 to simulate the conversation between a patient and a psychotherapist. Like any other primitive AI technology of its time, ELIZA followed a set of explicitly programmed rules. For example, in response to any sentence uttered by the patient in the form of "I am —-" (e.g., "I am sad" or "I am anxious"), ELIZA was programmed to reply "how long have you been —-?" regardless of the meaning of the word or phrase in the blank space. This type of rule-based programming remained the dominant approach to AI for more than a decade as the experts at the time believed that "there is no reason, for example, why a team of specialists in some area, such as internal medicine, could not lay out as complicated a set of rules as they need for producing diagnoses from sets of symptoms" [3]. However, by 1980s, it became apparent that the field of medicine was "so broad and complex that it is difficult, if not impossible, to capture the relevant information in rules" [4]. As a result, the AI community embraced a radically different approach called machine learning in which computers, rather than being explicitly programmed with rules, leverage data to derive their own rules.

As a computational framework for learning from data, machine learning has produced ground-breaking advances in medicine as well as many other fields of science and technology. A special breed of machine learning models (called deep learning) now rival human experts at performing certain clinical tasks including image-based diagnosis of skin cancer (see e.g., [5]). Using this particular application as a working example, in the next section, we introduce the standard machine learning pipeline. Later in the chapter, we discuss the basic taxonomy of machine learning problems and present a host of other applications of this powerful technology in medicine.

The Machine Learning Pipeline

In this section, we describe the procedures involved in building a prototypical machine learning system to perform a routine dermatology assessment: distinguishing between benign and malignant skin lesions. Working through this example will allow us to introduce the machine learning pipeline (in its most basic form) and describe the fundamental concepts underlying it.

Data Collection

Since machine learning is built on the principle of learning from data, it makes intuitive sense that collecting data constitutes the first step in the machine learning pipeline. In our dermatology example, the data to be collected is in the form of images of skin lesions, each labeled as either *benign* or *malignant* by a human

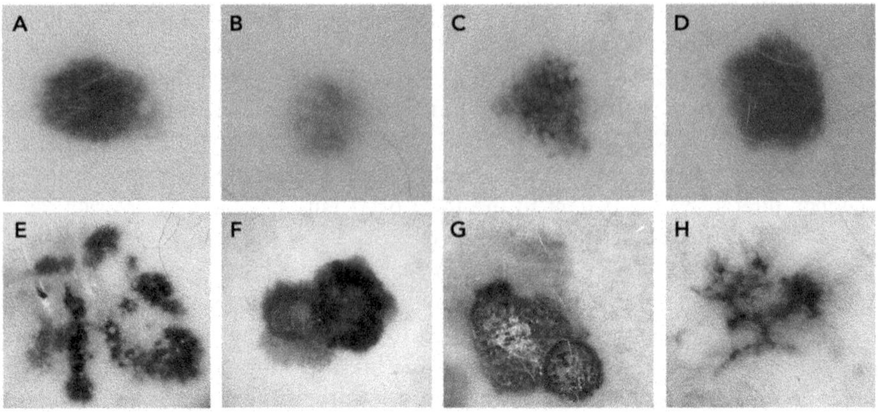

Fig. 1.2 A small classification dataset consisting of four benign lesions (top row) and four malignant lesions (bottom row). The images shown in this figure were taken from the international skin imaging collaboration (ISIC) dataset [6]

expert, e.g., a dermatologist. It is important to note that while dermatologists are trained to detect various types of skin cancers visually (even in the early stages of the disease), the definitive diagnosis of cancer is only made following histopathological examination of the biopsied lesion in the lab. In the jargon of machine learning, pathologists provide the *ground truth* for each sample, and the kind of task where we teach a computer to distinguish between two types or *classes* of data (here, benign and malignant lesions) is called *classification*. In Fig. 1.2, we show a small *dataset* for the task at hand that consists of eight samples or *data points*.

As a general rule, we want the training dataset to be as large and diverse as possible because more examples give the machine learning system more experience. In practice, machine learning datasets can include millions of data points.

Feature Design

To differentiate between benign and malignant lesions, dermatologists consider a combination of different attributes of the lesion including its morphology, color, and size.[3] These attributes are called *features* in the language of machine learning. It is well known that malignant lesions generally have less symmetric shapes and

[3] Other factors such as the patient's life style, over-exposure to UV light, and familial history of the disease also play a role in guiding the physician toward a cancer diagnosis. Nonetheless, we build our machine learning system using the lesion's appearance alone.

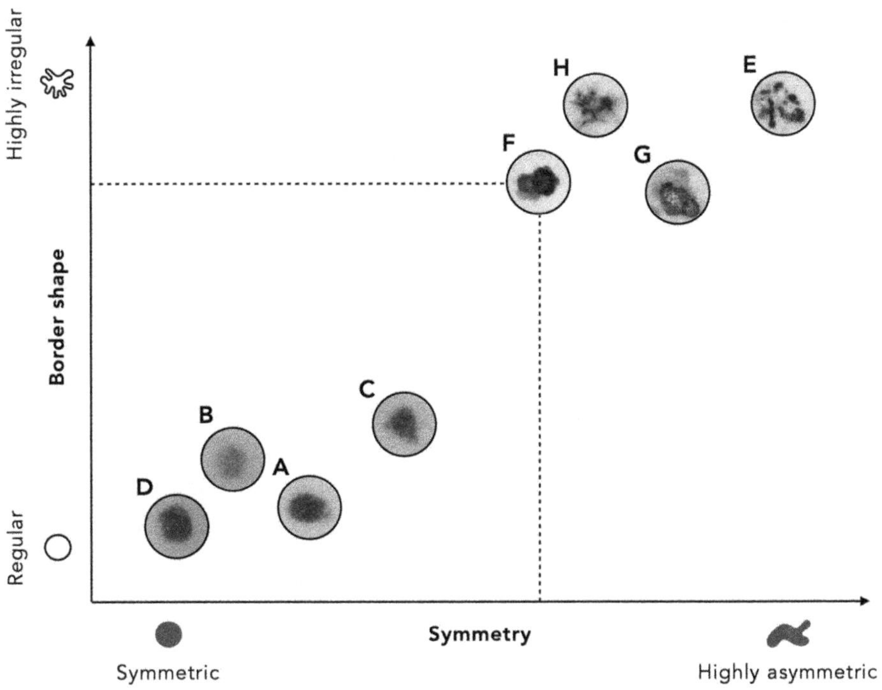

Fig. 1.3 Feature space representation of the dataset shown previously in Fig. 1.2. Here the horizontal and vertical axes represent the *symmetry* and *border shape* features, respectively. The fact that the benign and malignant lesions lie in distinct regions of the feature space reflects a good choice of features

more irregular borders compared to benign nevi, as reflected in the small dataset shown in Fig. 1.2. While quantifying these qualitative features is not a trivial task, for the sake of simplicity, suppose we can easily extract the following two features from each image in our dataset: first, *symmetry* ranging from perfectly symmetric to highly asymmetric, and second, *border shape* ranging from perfectly regular to highly irregular. With this choice of features, each image can be represented in a two-dimensional *feature space*, depicted in Fig. 1.3, by just two numbers: a number measuring the lesion's symmetry that determines the horizontal position of the image and another number capturing the lesion's border shape that determines its vertical position in the feature space.

Designing proper features is crucial to the overall success of a classification system. Quality features allow for the two classes of data to be well-separated in the feature space, as is the case with our choice of features in Fig. 1.3.

Model Training

With data represented in a carefully designed feature space, the problem of distinguishing between benign and malignant lesions reduces to separating the data points in each class with a line. In the parlance of machine learning, this line is referred to as a *classification model* (or *classifier* for short), and the process of finding an optimal classification model is called *model training*. Once a classifier is trained, the feature space will be divided into two subspaces falling on either side of the classifier. Figure 1.4 shows a trained linear classifier that divides the feature space into benign and malignant subspaces. Notice, how this classifier provides a simple rule for distinguishing between benign and malignant lesions: when the feature representation of a lesion lies below the line (in the blue region), it will be classified as benign, and likewise any feature representation that falls above the line (in the yellow region) will be classified as malignant.

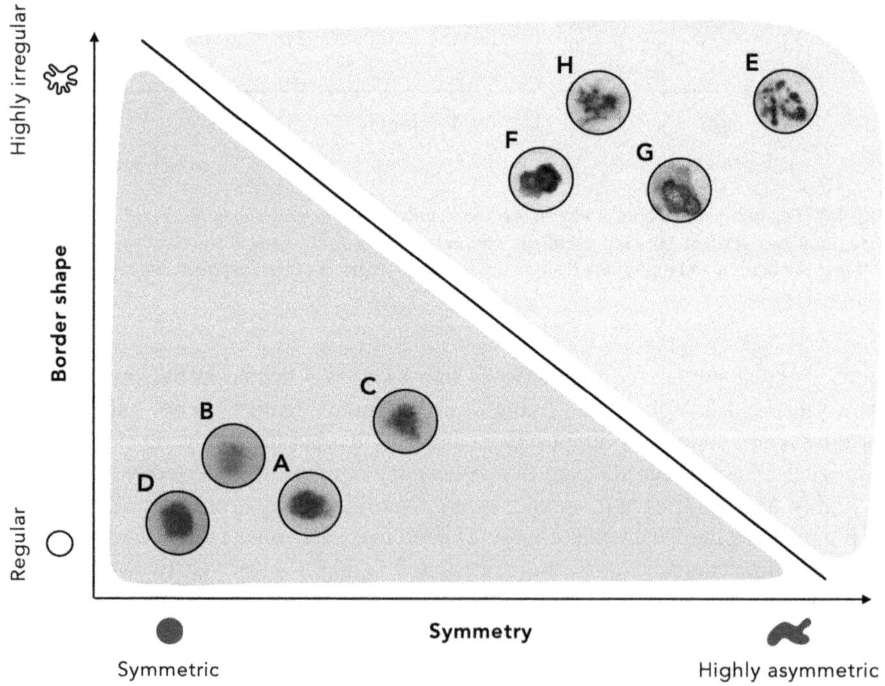

Fig. 1.4 Model training involves finding an appropriate line that separates the two classes of data in the feature space. The linear classifier shown in black provides a computational rule for distinguishing between benign and malignant lesions. A lesion is classified as benign if its feature representation lies below the line (in the blue region) and malignant if the feature representation lies above it (in the yellow region)

Model Testing

The classification model shown in Fig. 1.4 does an excellent job at separating the feature representations of the benign and malignant lesions, with no data point being classified incorrectly. This, however, should not give us too much confidence about the classifier's efficacy. The real test of a classifier is when it can *generalize* what it has learned to new or previously unseen instances of the data. This evaluation is done via the process of *model testing*. To test a classification model, we must collect a new batch of data, called *testing data*, as shown in Fig. 1.5. Clearly, there should be no overlap between the testing dataset and the set of data used previously during training, which from now on we refer to as the *training dataset*.

The model testing process begins with obtaining the feature representation of each image in the testing dataset using the previously designed set of features (i.e., symmetry and border shape). With both features extracted, we then find the position of each testing image in the feature space relative to the trained linear classifier. As illustrated in Fig. 1.6, all four benign lesions fall below the line in the blue region and are thus classified correctly as benign by the classifier. Similarly, two of the four malignant lesions fall above the line in the yellow region and, as a result, are classified correctly as malignant. However, two malignant lesions (namely, the data points `M` and `N`) end up on the wrong side of the line in the blue region and are therefore *misclassified* as benign by the classifier.

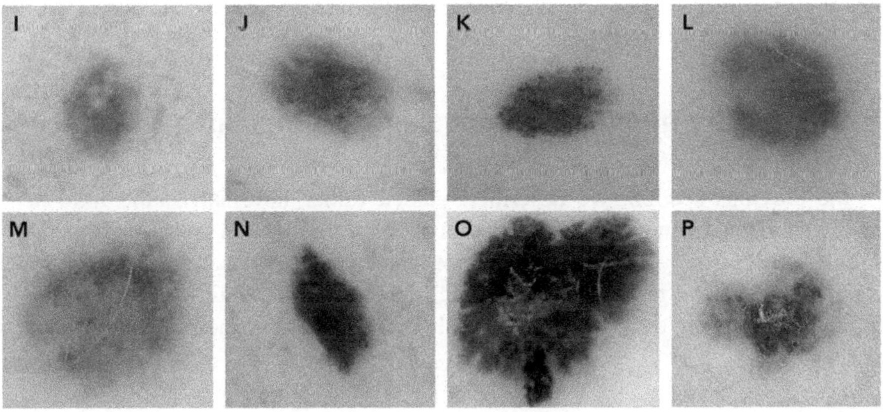

Fig. 1.5 A testing dataset of benign (top row) and malignant (bottom row) skin lesions. The training dataset illustrated in Fig. 1.2 and the testing dataset illustrated here must not have any data point in common. The images shown in this figure were taken from the international skin imaging collaboration (ISIC) dataset [6]

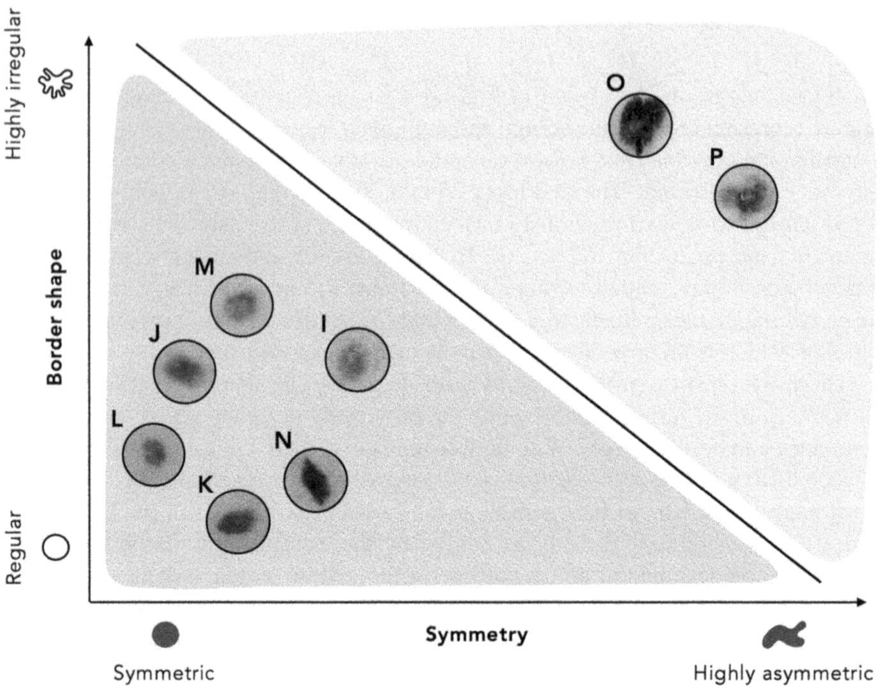

Fig. 1.6 The feature representations of two of the eight testing data points end up on the wrong side of the linear classifier. As a result, these two malignant lesions (M and N) will be classified incorrectly as benign by the model

A Deeper Dive into the Machine Learning Pipeline

In the previous section, we described—albeit rather informally—the four steps involved in developing a prototypical skin cancer classification system. These steps, summarized visually in Fig. 1.7, include data collection, feature design, model training, and model testing. With this high-level understanding, we are now ready to delve deeper into each step of the pipeline and discuss further relevant ideas and concepts.

Revisiting Data Collection

Data is the fuel that powers machine learning, and as such "the more is always the merrier" when it comes to data. However, in practice, there are often cost, security, and patient privacy concerns that can each severely limit data availability. In such circumstances, proper rationing of the available data between the training and testing sets becomes important.

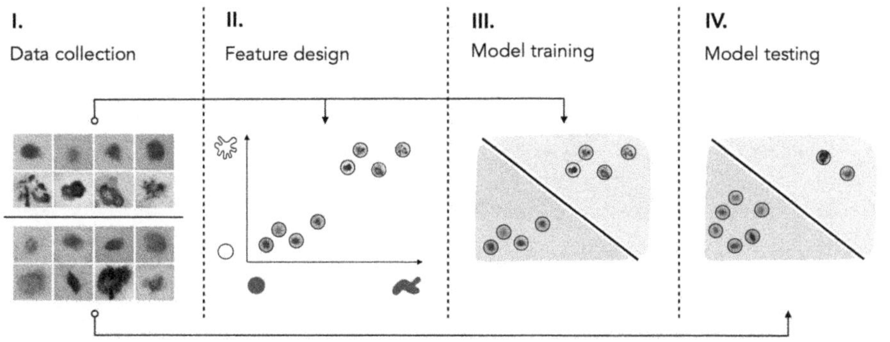

Fig. 1.7 The schematic summary of the classification pipeline discussed in Sect. "The Machine Learning Pipeline"

There is no precise rule for what portion of a given dataset should be set aside for testing. On one hand, we want the training set to be as large as possible so that the classifier can learn from a wide array of data samples. On the other hand, a large and diverse testing set ensures that the trained model can reliably classify previously unseen instances. As a rule of thumb, between 10% and 30% of the whole data is typically assigned at random to the testing set. Generally speaking, the percentage of the original data that may be assigned to the testing set increases as the size of the data increases. The intuition for this is that when the data is plentiful, the training set still accurately represents the underlying phenomenon of interest, even after removal of a relatively large set of testing data. Conversely, with smaller datasets, we usually take a smaller percentage for testing since the relatively larger training set needs to retain what little information of the underlying phenomenon was captured by the original data, and as a result, smaller amounts of data can be spared for testing.

Revisiting Feature Design

In assessing skin lesions for potential malignancies, dermatologists sometimes apply the so-called ABCDE rule: an abbreviation for the asymmetry, border, color, diameter, and evolving or changing appearance of the lesion. This rule was the basis for choosing symmetry and border shape as features in Sect. "The Machine Learning Pipeline". Unfortunately, we cannot always rely on our prior clinical knowledge to design features since it may be incomplete—or even non-existent—depending on the task at hand. Therefore, it would be highly convenient and desirable if we could circumvent the feature design step altogether by using the raw input data directly to train the classification model. Let us take a moment to explore this option more thoroughly.

The data for the skin cancer classification task comprises color images of size 512×512. A color image is essentially a superimposition of three mono-color

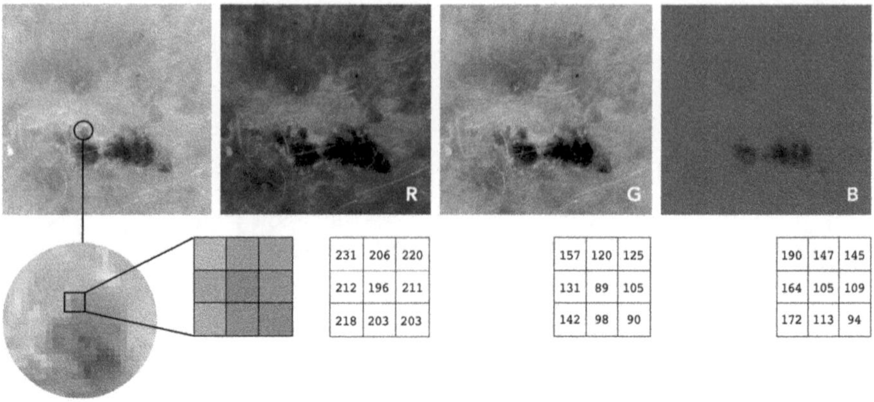

Fig. 1.8 A color image is made up of three color bands or channels: red (R), green (G), and blue (B). Every pixel in a color image can therefore be represented as a list of three integers (one for each channel) with an intensity value ranging from 0 to 255

channels as illustrated in Fig. 1.8. Multiplying the total number of pixels (i.e., 512^2) by the number of color channels per pixel (i.e., 3), we arrive at a number close to 800,000. This would be the dimension of the feature space if we were to use raw pixel values as features!

Ultra-high-dimensional spaces like this cause an undesired phenomenon called the *curse of dimensionality*. To provide an intuitive description of this phenomenon, we begin with a simple one-dimensional space and work our way up from there to higher dimensions. Suppose we aim to understand what goes on inside a one-dimensional space (i.e., a line). We place a series of sensors on this line, each at a distance of d from its neighboring sensors. Clearly, the smaller the value of d the larger the number of required sensors and the more fine-grained our understanding of the space under study. Setting d to a fixed pre-determined value, as shown in the left panel of Fig. 1.9, we need 3 sensors to cover a line segment of length $2d$. Now let us move up one dimension. As illustrated in the middle panel of Fig. 1.9, in a two-dimensional space (i.e., a plane), we will need 9 sensors to cover a $2d \times 2d$ area with the same level of resolution (or granularity). Similarly, in a three-dimensional space, we will need a total of 27 sensors, as illustrated in the right panel of Fig. 1.9. Extrapolating this pattern into higher dimensions, 3^N sensors are needed in a general N-dimensional space. In other words, the number of sensors grows *exponentially* with the dimension of the space.

Data points are essentially like sensors since they relay to us useful information about the space they lie in. The larger the number of data points (sensors) the fuller our understanding of the feature space. The problem is as the dimension N of the feature space increases we need exponentially more data points to perform classification effectively—something that is not feasible when N is extremely large.

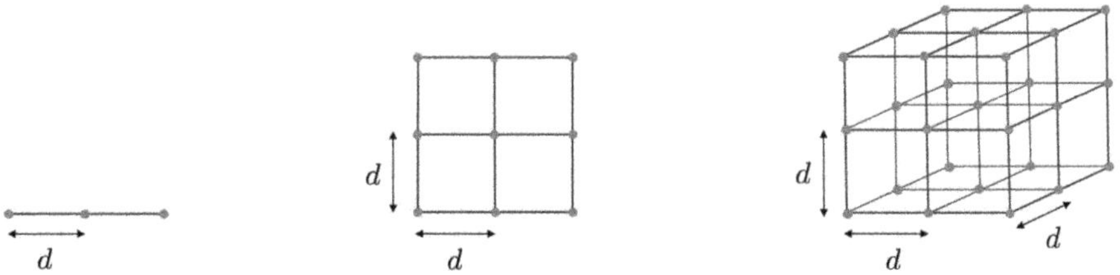

Fig. 1.9 The number of sensors (shown as red dots) that we must place so that each is at a distance of d from its neighboring sensors grows exponentially with the dimension of the space. This exponential growth behavior is commonly referred to as the curse of dimensionality

We just saw how "the curse of dimensionality" practically prohibits the use of raw pixel values as features.[4] The good news is that, as we will see later in the book, deep learning allows for the automatic learning of the features from the data. In fact, in a typical deep learning classification system, the *feature design* and *model training* steps are combined into one step so that both the features and the classifier are learned jointly from the data.

Revisiting Model Training

As discussed previously in Sect. "The Machine Learning Pipeline", training of a linear classifier boils down to finding a line that divides the feature space into two regions: one region per each class of data. Here we discuss what the process of finding this line actually entails in greater detail.

Any line in a two-dimensional space can be characterized by three parameters: two *slope* parameters measuring the line's orientation in each dimension, as well as a *bias* or offset parameter. Denoting the two dimensions by x_1 and x_2, the corresponding slope parameters by w_1 and w_2, and the bias parameter by w_0, the equation of a line can be written formally as

$$w_0 + w_1 x_1 + w_2 x_2 = 0. \quad (1.1)$$

For example, setting $w_0 = 0$, $w_1 = 1$, and $w_2 = -1$ results in a line with the equation $x_1 - x_2 = 0$, which goes through the origin while forming a 45° angle with both the horizontal and vertical axes. Of all possible values for w_0, w_1, and w_2,

[4] Even if the extremely large dimension of the feature space were not an issue, by using raw pixel values as features, we would disregard the valuable information that can be inferred from the location of each pixel in the image. In Chap. 7, we will study a family of deep learning models called *convolutional neural networks* that are specifically designed to leverage the spatial correlations present in imaging data.

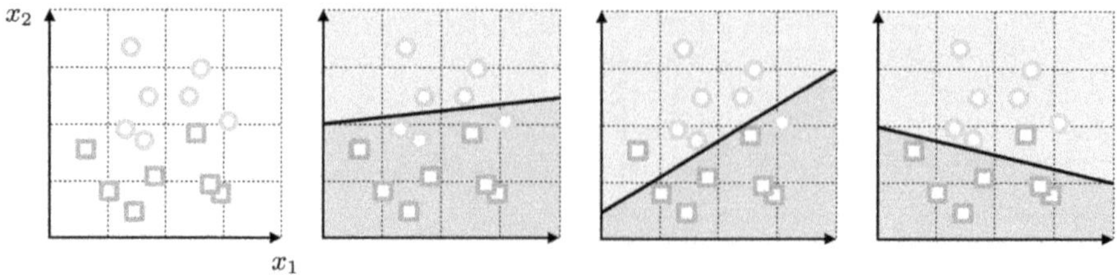

Fig. 1.10 (First panel) The feature space representation of a toy classification dataset consisting of two classes of data: blue squares and yellow circles. (Second panel) The line defined by the parameters $(w_0, w_1, w_2) = (16, 1, -8)$ classifies three yellow circles incorrectly, hence $g(16, 1, -8) = 3$. (Third panel) The line defined by the parameters $(w_0, w_1, w_2) = (4, 5, -8)$ misclassifies one yellow circle and one blue square, hence $g(4, 5, -8) = 2$. (Fourth panel) The line defined by the parameters $(w_0, w_1, w_2) = (-8, 1, 4)$ classifies only a single blue square incorrectly, hence $g(-8, 1, 4) = 1$

we look for those resulting in a line that separates the two classes of data as best as possible. More precisely, we want to set the line parameters so as to minimize the number of errors or misclassifications made by the classifier. We can express this idea mathematically by denoting by $g(w_0, w_1, w_2)$ a function that takes a particular set of line parameters as input and returns as output the number of classification errors made by the classifier $w_0 + w_1x_1 + w_2x_2 = 0$. In Fig. 1.10, we show three different settings of (w_0, w_1, w_2) for a toy classification dataset, resulting in three distinct classifiers and three different values of g.

The function g is commonly referred to as a *cost function* or *error function* in the machine learning terminology. We aim to *minimize* this function by finding *optimal* values for w_0, w_1, and w_2, denoted, respectively, by $w_0^\star$, $w_1^\star$, and $w_2^\star$, such that

$$g(w_0^\star, w_1^\star, w_2^\star) \leq g(w_0, w_1, w_2) \tag{1.2}$$

for all values of w_0, w_1, and w_2. For example, for the toy classification dataset shown in Fig. 1.10, we have that $w_0^\star = -8$, $w_1^\star = 1$, and $w_2^\star = 4$. This corresponds to a minimum cost value of $g(w_0^\star, w_1^\star, w_2^\star) = 1$, which is the smallest number of errors attainable by any linear classifier on this particular set of data. The process of determining the optimal parameter values for a given cost function is referred to as *mathematical optimization*.

Note that unlike the skin cancer classification dataset shown in Fig. 1.4, the toy dataset in Fig. 1.10 is not *linearly separable*, meaning that no linear model can be found to classify it without error. This type of data is commonplace in practice and requires more sophisticated *nonlinear* classification models such as the ones shown in Fig. 1.11. In the second, third, and fourth panels of this figure, we show an instance of a polynomial, decision tree, and artificial neural network classifier, respectively. These are the three most popular families of nonlinear classification models, with the latter family being the focus of our study in Chaps. 6 and 7.

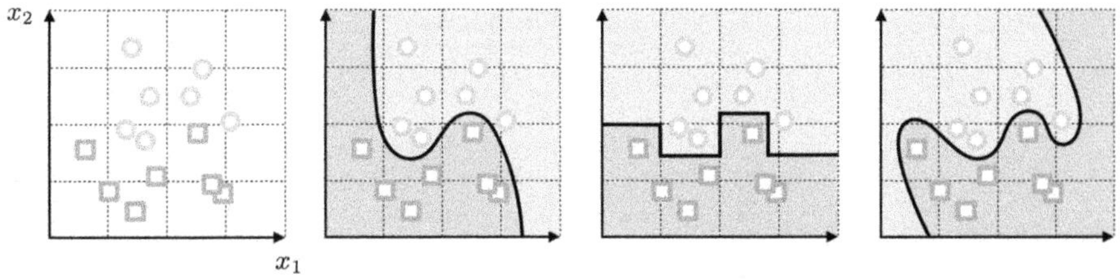

Fig. 1.11 (First panel) The toy classification dataset shown originally in Fig. 1.10. (Second panel) A polynomial classifier. (Third panel) A decision tree classifier. (Fourth panel) A neural network classifier. Each of the *nonlinear* classifiers shown here is capable of separating the two classes of data perfectly

Revisiting Model Testing

By evaluating the performance of the linear classifier shown in Fig. 1.6, we can see that it correctly classifies six of the eight samples in the testing dataset. Dividing the first number by the second gives a widely used quality metric for classification called *accuracy*, defined as

$$\text{accuracy} = \frac{\text{number of correctly classified data points in the testing set}}{\text{total number of data points in the testing set}}. \tag{1.3}$$

Based on the definition given above, this metric always ranges between 0 and 1, with larger values of it being more desirable. In our example, accuracy $= \frac{6}{8} = 0.75$.

While accuracy does provide a useful metric for the overall performance of a classifier, it does not distinguish between the misclassification of a benign lesion as malignant (type I error) and the misclassification of a malignant lesion as benign (type II error). Since this distinction is particularly important in the context of medicine, two additional metrics are often used to report classification results. Denoting the malignant class as *positive* (for cancer) and the benign class as *negative*, the two metrics of *sensitivity* and *specificity* are defined, respectively, as

$$\text{sensitivity} = \frac{\text{number of positive data points correctly classified as positive}}{\text{total number of data points in the positive class}}$$

$$\text{specificity} = \frac{\text{number of negative data points correctly classified as negative}}{\text{total number of data points in the negative class}}. \tag{1.4}$$

As with accuracy, both sensitivity and specificity always range between 0 and 1, with larger values of them being more desirable. In our example, sensitivity $= \frac{2}{4} = 0.5$ and specificity $= \frac{4}{4} = 1$.

All three classification metrics introduced so far (i.e., accuracy, sensitivity, and specificity) can be expressed more compactly and elegantly using the so-called

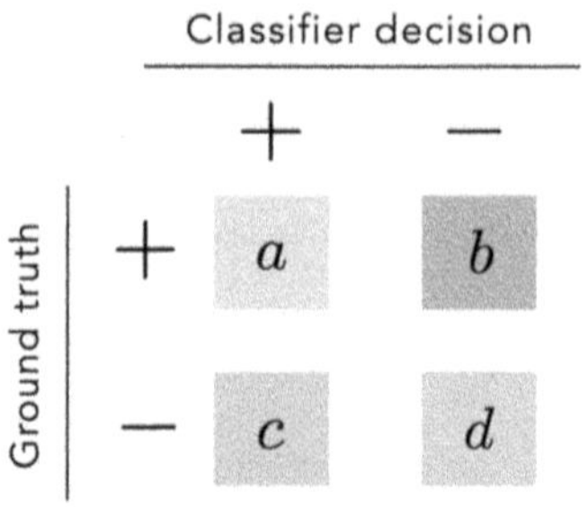

Fig. 1.12 A confusion matrix illustrated. Here a is the number of positive data points classified correctly as positive, b is the number of positive data points classified incorrectly as negative, c is the number of negative data points classified incorrectly as positive, and d is the number of negative data points classified correctly as negative

confusion matrix. As illustrated in Fig. 1.12, a confusion matrix is a simple look-up table where classification results are broken down by *ground truth* (across rows) and *classifier decision* (across columns).

Using the confusion matrix, we can rewrite the classification metrics in Eqs. (1.3) and (1.4) more succinctly as

$$\text{accuracy} = \frac{a+d}{a+b+c+d}, \quad \text{sensitivity} = \frac{a}{a+b}, \quad \text{specificity} = \frac{d}{c+d}. \tag{1.5}$$

In addition to the metrics in Eq. (1.5), a number of other classification metrics can be calculated using the confusion matrix, among which *balanced accuracy*, *precision*, and F-*score* (as defined below) are more frequently used in the literature.

$$\text{balanced accuracy} = \frac{\frac{a}{a+b}+\frac{d}{c+d}}{2}, \quad \text{precision} = \frac{a}{a+c}, \quad \text{F-score} = \frac{2a}{2a+b+c}. \tag{1.6}$$

The Machine Learning Taxonomy

In Sects. "The Machine Learning Pipeline" and "A Deeper Dive into the Machine Learning Pipeline", we motivated the introduction of the machine learning pipeline using image-based diagnosis of skin cancer (see, e.g., [5]). This is just one of many diagnostic tasks where machine learning has achieved human-level accuracy. Another examples include diagnosis of diabetic retinopathy using retinal fundus photographs (see e.g., [7]), diagnosis of breast cancer using mammograms (see e.g., [8]), diagnosis of lung cancer using chest computed tomography (CT) images (see e.g., [9]), diagnosis of bladder cancer using cystoscopy images (see e.g., [10]), and many more (Fig. 1.13).

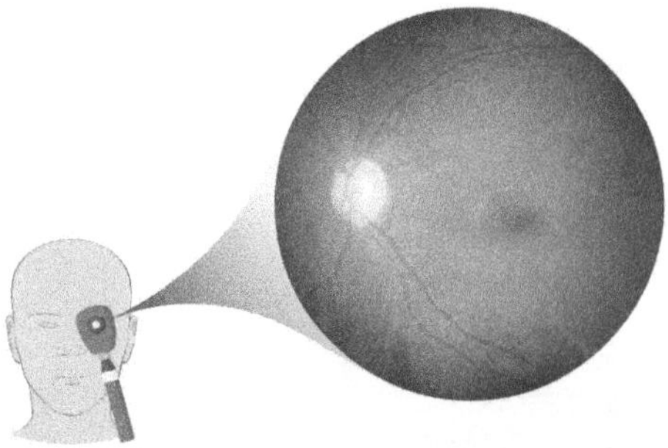

Fig. 1.13 A retinal fundus image captures important structures in the eye. This imaging modality is typically used for diagnosis and monitoring of diabetic retinopathy, hypertensive retinopathy, macular degeneration, etc.

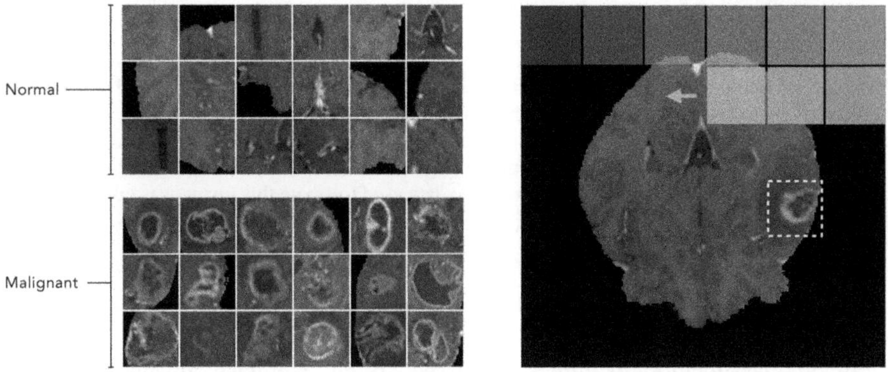

Fig. 1.14 (Left panel) A sample training dataset for the task of brain tumor localization. (Right panel) To determine if any tumors are present in a given brain MRI, a small window is scanned across it from top to bottom. If the image content inside the window is deemed malignant by a trained classifier, its location will be marked by a bounding box. The images used to create this figure were taken from the brain tumor image segmentation (BRATS) dataset [11]

In addition to medical diagnosis, the classification framework also lends itself well to *localization* tasks where we aim to automatically identify the location of a specific object of interest (e.g., a tumor) in a set of medical images (e.g., MRI scans of the brain). The same kind of classification pipeline we studied previously in the case of skin cancer classification can be utilized to solve localization problems. For example, a classifier can be trained on a dataset containing images of tumors as well as normal tissues of the brain (see Fig. 1.14; left panel). Once the training is complete, tumors are sought after in a new MRI scan by sliding a small window across it. At each location of the sliding window, the image content inside it tested to see which side of the classifier it lies on. If it lies on the "tumor side" of the classifier, the content is classified as a tumor, and a bounding box is drawn around it to highlight its location (see Fig. 1.14; right panel).

The classification framework can also be utilized to make predictions about medical events that have a "future component." For example, prediction of 1-year or 5-year survival in cancer patients is naturally a classification problem, having only two possible outcomes (or classes). Predicting whether a patient will be re-

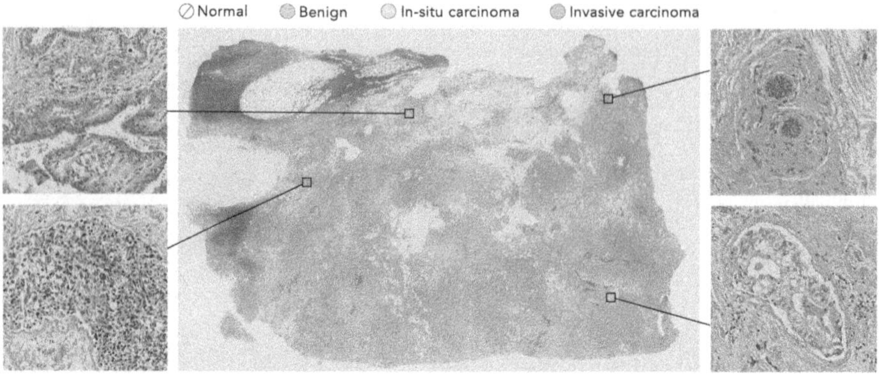

Fig. 1.15 (Middle panel) A whole-slide image of breast tissue. In addition to normal regions that make up the vast majority of the slides, there are multiple benign, in situ carcinoma, and invasive carcinoma regions in this image that are highlighted in green, yellow, and blue, respectively. (Side panels) Four 800 × 800 patches, each representing one of the four classes in the data, are blown up in the side panels for better visualization. The data used to create this image was taken from the breast cancer histology (BACH) dataset [13]

admitted to the hospital shortly following discharge is another problem of interest in healthcare that can be cast as classification.

In all classification examples discussed so far, we have always sought to distinguish between two classes of data (e.g., benign versus malignant skin lesions). Because of this binary nature of the output, the problem solved in each case is more precisely referred to as *binary* or *two-class classification*. However, classification can be applied more generally to medical tasks where there are more than just two classes that we wish to distinguish, e.g., tumor grading/staging. In Fig. 1.15, we show a whole-slide image of breast tissue in a patient with carcinoma wherein each region of the image is marked as either normal, benign, in situ carcinoma, or invasive carcinoma by an expert pathologist. In this case, a *multi-class* classifier can be trained to segment the entire image automatically into one of the four aforementioned classes. Note that while the biopsied sample shown in Fig. 1.15 is only a few centimeters long in width and height, its high-resolution whole-slide image consists of approximately 2.4 billion pixels! A time-consuming aspect of a pathologist's job is to carefully examine each and every spot in this giga-pixel image in search of malignancies. In the early stages of the disease, there may only be a few cancerous cells present in the whole slide that can easily be missed during visual inspection. This arduous process can be streamlined using a multi-class classifier trained to direct the attention of the pathologist to the irregular regions of the slide.

Sometimes the variables we wish to predict using medical data are *continuous* in nature, e.g., systolic blood pressure, body mass index (BMI), age, etc. These variables can take on *any* value within a given range. For example, 88 mmHg, 124 mmHg, and 165 mmHg are all valid blood pressure values. Similarly, 17 kg/m^2, 24.1 kg/m^2, and 32.8 kg/m^2 are possible BMI values. In this regard, continuous variables are intrinsically different from their *discrete* counterparts such as blood type or tumor stage that always take on a few pre-determined values: {`O`, `A`, `B`, `AB`} for blood type, and {`I`, `II`, `III`, `IV`} for tumor stage. In the nomenclature of machine learning, the task of predicting a continuous output from input data is called *regression*. It is interesting, and somewhat surprising, to note that all the continuous variables mentioned here (i.e., blood pressure, BMI, and age) can be predicted to varying degrees of accuracy [12] using retinal scans (like the one shown in Fig. 1.13).

In all problem instances we have seen so far, there is always a discrete-valued (in the case of classification) or continuous-valued (in the case of regression) *output* that we wish to predict using *input* data. A machine learning classifier or regressor tries to learn this input/output relationship using data labeled by a human *supervisor*. Because of this reliance on labeled data, both classification and regression are considered *supervised learning* schemes. Another category of machine learning problems called *unsupervised learning* deals with learning from the *input* data alone. In what follows, we briefly introduce two fundamental problems in this category: *clustering* and *dimension reduction*.

The objective of *clustering* is to identify groups or clusters of input data points that are similar to each other. For example, in the left panel of Fig. 1.16, we show a gene expression microarray that is a two-dimensional matrix with 33 rows (patient samples) and 20 columns (genes). Each square on this 33×20 grid represents the color-coded expression level of a particular gene in a tissue sample collected from a patient with leukemia. In the right panel of Fig. 1.16, we show the results of clustering the rows and columns of this microarray data. As can been seen, the genes across the columns of the microarray form two equally sized clusters. Similarly, the patients across the rows of the microarray are clustered into two groups of sizes 22 and 11, respectively. Automatic identification of such gene and patient clusters can lead to the discovery of new gene targets for drug therapy (see e.g., [14, 15]).

Modern-day medical datasets can be extremely high-dimensional. This is both a blessing and a curse. High-resolution pathology and radiology scans allow physicians to see minute details that could lead to early diagnosis of disease. Similarly, large-scale RNA sequencing datasets give researchers the ability to detect genetic variations at the level of the nucleotide. However, this level of resolution comes at a price. Recall from our discussion of the curse of dimensionality in Sect. "A Deeper Dive into the Machine Learning Pipeline" that as the dimension of the data grows, we need exponentially larger datasets (in terms of the number of data points). When acquiring such large amounts of data is not feasible, reducing the dimension of data—if possible—will be crucial for training effective models.

Geometrically speaking, in order to reduce the dimension of a dataset, we must find a lower-dimensional representation (sometimes called a *manifold*) for the data points in their original high-dimensional space. This general idea is illustrated in Fig. 1.17 using an overly simplistic two-dimensional dataset consisting of eight data points. As depicted in the left panel of the figure, each data point in this two-dimensional space is generally represented by two numbers—a and b—indicating its horizontal and vertical coordinates. However, if the data points happen to lie on

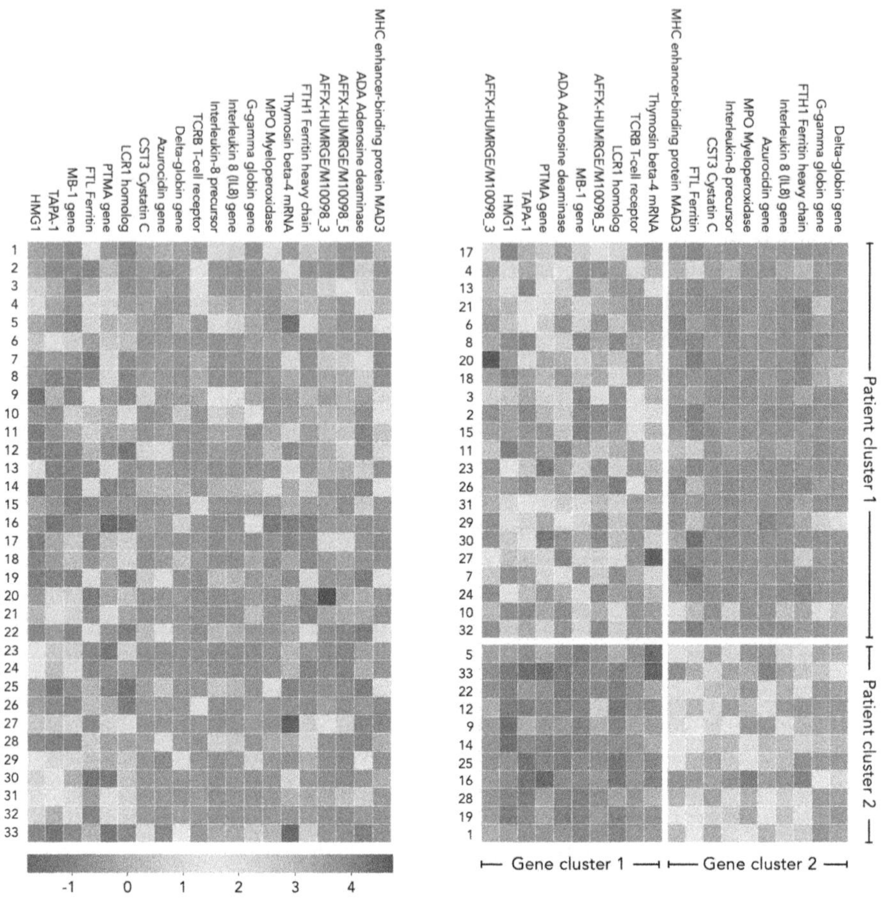

Fig. 1.16 (Left panel) A gene expression microarray of 20 genes (across columns) and 33 patients with leukemia (across rows). (Right panel) Clustering of this data reveals two groups of similar patients and two groups of similar genes. The data used to create this figure was taken from [16]

a circular manifold and we are able to uncover it (as shown in the right panel of Fig. 1.17), each data point can then be represented using one number only: the angle θ between the horizontal axis and the line segment connecting the data point to the origin. This brings the dimension of the original dataset down from two to one.

Dimension reduction techniques operate under the assumption that the original high-dimensional data lies (approximately) in a lower-dimensional subspace and that we can discover this subspace relatively easily. Sometimes this assumption does not hold. In such cases, we can take an alternative approach to combat the curse of dimensionality. Rather than reducing the dimension of data, we increase the size of data by creating synthetic data points. Figure 1.18 shows a set of real images of skin lesions along with a batch of synthetic but realistic-looking lesions generated to augment the size of the original data. It is worth noting that the number of

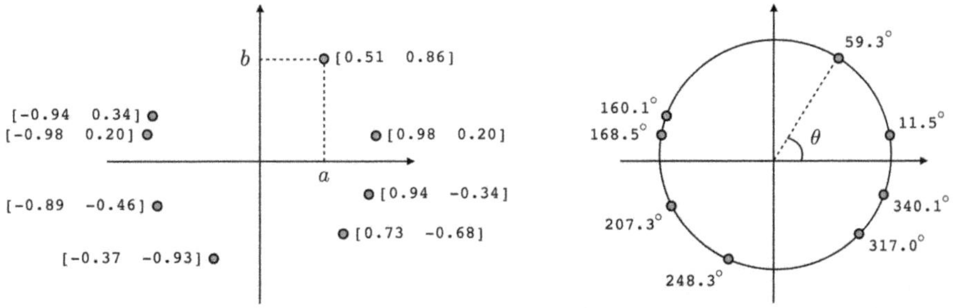

Fig. 1.17 (Left panel) A toy two-dimensional dataset with eight data points shown in red. Each data point is represented by a pair of numbers a and b indicating its location relative to the horizontal and vertical axes. (Right panel) Because this particular set of data happens to lie on a circular manifold, the location of each data point can be encoded using the angle θ alone. Note that the discovery of this circular manifold was key in reducing the dimension of this dataset from two to one

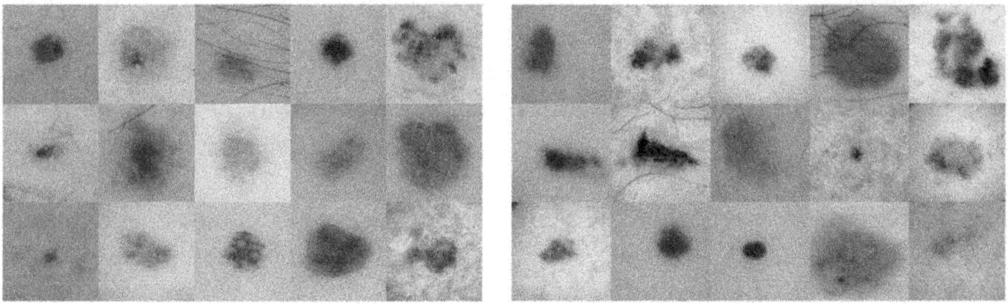

Fig. 1.18 (Left panel) A collection of *real* skin lesions taken from the international skin imaging collaboration (ISIC) dataset [6]. (Right panel) A collection of *fake* lesions generated using machine learning [18]

supervised applications of machine learning in medicine dwarfs that of unsupervised applications. Moreover, the study of the type of models[5] that could generate the data in Fig. 1.18 requires a prerequisite knowledge of machine learning and deep learning which this book aims to provide. For these reasons, we have left the discussion of unsupervised learning models out of this introductory book and refer the interested reader to more advanced treatments of subject (see e.g., [17]).

Another machine learning strategy that may be employed when the size of data is smaller than desired is called *transfer learning*. Using this approach, we can transfer the knowledge gained while solving one problem to a different but related problem. Transfer learning can be especially useful when dealing with new phenomena for which no historical data is available. For example, during the outbreak of the COVID-19 pandemic, researchers leveraged abundant chest X-ray images of patients with other respiratory disorders to train a deep learning model for

[5] Generative adversarial networks.

diagnosing COVID-19 using transfer learning (see, e.g., [19]). We discuss transfer learning in more detail in Chap. 7.

In every machine learning problem, we have seen so far a model is trained to make a *single* decision for which it receives an *immediate* reward. For example, presented with an image of a skin lesion, a skin cancer classifier has only one decision to make: is the lesion benign or malignant? If the classifier answers this question correctly, its accuracy score will improve as a result. *Reinforcement learning* extends this general framework to more complex scenarios where a computer agent is trained to make a *sequence* of decisions in pursuit of a *long-term* goal. To better understand this distinction, consider the game of chess: a computer trained to play chess must make a series of decisions—in the form of chess-piece moves—with the long-term goal of check-mating its opponent. Each decision is called an *action* in the context of reinforcement learning. "Moving the queen up two squares" is an example of an action. Note, however, that depending on the *state* of the chessboard, this action may or may not be allowed. For example, if an enemy piece is on the square right above the queen, she must eliminate it first before being able to move to her desired location. In the parlance of reinforcement learning, a *state* is a variable that communicates characteristic information about the problem environment (e.g., the location of each piece on the board) to the computer agent. Reinforcement learning problems are inherently *dynamic* because every action taken by the agent changes the state of the environment.

In medicine, reinforcement learning has been applied to devising treatment policies in diabetes [20], cancer [21], and sepsis [22]. For example, to achieve the *long-term goal* of full recovery from sepsis in an intensive care unit, a computer agent can learn to take appropriate *actions* depending on the patient's *state*. The action space of this problem includes administering antibiotics, administering intravenous fluids, placing the patient on mechanical ventilation, etc. Taking each of these actions leads to a change (for better or worse) in the patient's state captured via their vital measurements and lab tests (see, e.g., [23]). We will study reinforcement learning in Chap. 8.

Problems

1.1 Strategies to Combat the Curse of Dimensionality

Suppose that a training set of data consists of P data points lying in an N-dimensional space. The curse of dimensionality dictates that the fraction $\frac{P}{N}$ should ideally be as large as possible for effective training of machine learning models. Name two strategies we discussed in Sect. "The Machine Learning Taxonomy" that can be employed to increase the value of $\frac{P}{N}$.

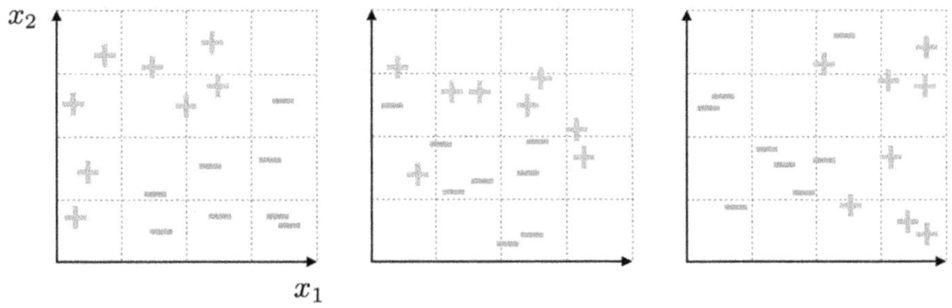

Fig. 1.19 Figure associated with Exercises 1.2 and 1.3. See text for details

1.2 Classification by Trial and Error: Part I

Three toy classification datasets are shown in Fig. 1.19. Using an object with a straight edge (e.g., a ruler), try a range of different linear classifiers for each dataset, and find the one that produces the minimum number of errors or misclassifications.

(a) Report the parameters w_0, w_1, and w_2 for the optimal classifier you found in each case. Hint: See Eq. (1.1) and Fig. 1.10.
(b) Would this trial-and-error strategy work if the datasets were three-dimensional instead? What if they were four-dimensional?

1.3 Classification by Trial and Error: Part II

For each of the classifiers you found in Exercise 1.2:

(a) Form the confusion matrix.
(b) Calculate accuracy, sensitivity, and specificity.

1.4 True or False?

"*For any given training dataset regardless of its shape and size, there always exists a linear or nonlinear classifier that can separate the two classes of data perfectly*." Is this statement true or false? If true, prove it as rigorously as you can. Otherwise, provide a counter example.

1.5 Classification Quality Metrics

A linear classifier has achieved an accuracy score of 0.84, a sensitivity score of 0.8, and a specificity score of 0.9 on a binary classification dataset. In the absence of any information on the number of data points in each class, determine whether it is possible (or not) to calculate the classifier's:

(a) Balanced accuracy
(b) Precision
(c) F-score

1.6 Inequalities Involving Classification Quality Metrics

(a) Show that the values of accuracy and balanced accuracy as defined in Eqs. (1.5) and (1.6) always lie in between those of sensitivity and specificity.

(b) Show that the F-score always lies in between sensitivity and precision, but never exceeds their average.

1.7 Further Machine Learning and Deep Learning Applications

Based on the description provided below, determine what type of machine learning problem is solved in each case.

(a) Spampinato et al. [24] developed a machine learning system to predict skeletal bone age using hand X-ray images. Skeletal age assessment is a radiological procedure for determining bone age in children with growth and endocrine disorders. Ideally, the patient's skeletal age should be identical to their chronological age. Is this application an instance of binary classification, multi-class classification, regression, clustering, or dimension reduction? Explain.
(b) Miotto et al. [25] developed a deep learning system to derive a compact representation of patients' electronic health records (EHRs). The results obtained using this representation—dubbed "deep patient" by the authors—in a number of disease prediction tasks were better than those obtained by using the raw EHR data. Is this application an instance of binary classification, multi-class classification, regression, clustering, or dimension reduction? Explain.
(c) Hannun et al. [26] developed a deep learning system to detect multiple types of cardiac rhythms including the sinus rhythm and 10 different patterns of arrhythmia in single-lead electrocardiograms (ECGs), with the average F-score for their model exceeding that of the average cardiologist. Is this application an instance of binary classification, multi-class classification, regression, clustering, or dimension reduction? Explain.
(d) Razavian et al. [27] developed a deep learning system for patient risk stratification. Using lab results as input, their model was effective in predicting whether a patient would be diagnosed with a specific condition 3–15 months into the future from the time of prediction. Is this application an instance of binary classification, multi-class classification, regression, clustering, or dimension reduction? Explain.
(e) Tian et al. [28] developed a deep learning system to group individual cells together on the basis of transcriptome similarity using single-cell RNA sequencing (scRNA-seq) data. This type of data allows for fine-grained comparison of the transcriptomes at the level of the cell. Is this application an instance of binary classification, multi-class classification, regression, clustering, or dimension reduction? Explain.

References

1. Galilei G, Crew H, Salvio AD. Dialogues concerning two new sciences. New York: McGraw-Hill; 1963
2. Weizenbaum J. ELIZA: a computer program for the study of natural language communication between man and machine. Commun ACM. 1966;9(1):36–45

3. Galler BA. The value of computers to medicine. JAMA. 1960;174(17):2161–2
4. Schwartz WB, Patil RS, Szolovits P. Artificial intelligence in medicine – where do we stand? N Engl J Med. 1987;316:685–8
5. Esteva A, Kuprel B, Novoa R, et al. Dermatologist-level classification of skin cancer with deep neural networks. Nature. 2017;542:115–8
6. Rotemberg V, Kurtansky N, Betz-Stablein B, et al. A patient-centric dataset of images and metadata for identifying melanomas using clinical context. Nat Sci Data. 2021;8(34)
7. Gulshan V, Peng L, Coram M, et al. Development and validation of a deep learning algorithm for detection of diabetic retinopathy in retinal fundus photographs. JAMA. 2016;316(22):2402–10
8. McKinney SM, Sieniek M, Godbole V, et al. International evaluation of an AI system for breast cancer screening. Nature. 2020;577:89–94
9. Ardila D, Kiraly AP, Bharadwaj S, et al. End-to-end lung cancer screening with three-dimensional deep learning on low-dose chest computed tomography. Nat Med. 2019;25:954–61
10. Borhani S, Borhani R, Kajdacsy-Balla A. Artificial Intelligence: a promising frontier in bladder cancer diagnosis and outcome prediction. Crit Rev Oncol Hematol. 2022;171:103601. https://doi.org/10.1016/j.critrevonc.2022.103601
11. Menze BH, Jakab A, Bauer S, et al. The multimodal brain tumor image segmentation benchmark (BRATS). IEEE Trans Med Imag. 2015;34(10):1993–2024
12. Poplin R, Varadarajan AV, Blumer K, et al. Prediction of cardiovascular risk factors from retinal fundus photographs via deep learning. Nat Biomed Eng. 2018;2:158–64
13. Aresta G, Arajo T, Kwok S, et al. BACH: grand challenge on breast cancer histology images. Med Image Anal. 2019;56:122–39
14. Alizadeh A, Eisen M, Davis R, et al. Distinct types of diffuse large B-cell lymphoma identified by gene expression profiling. Nature. 2000;403:503–11
15. Chesnokov MS, Halasi M, Borhani S, et al. Novel FOXM1 inhibitor identified via gene network analysis induces autophagic FOXM1 degradation to overcome chemoresistance of human cancer cells. Cell Death Dis. 2021;12:704. https://doi.org/10.1038/s41419-021-03978-0
16. Golub TR, Slonim DK, Tamayo P, et al. Molecular classification of cancer: class discovery and class prediction by gene expression monitoring. Science. 1999;286(5439):531–37
17. Watt J, Borhani R, Katsaggelos AK. Machine learning refined: foundations, algorithms, and applications. Cambridge: Cambridge University Press; 2020
18. Baur C, Albarqouni S, Navab N. Generating highly realistic images of skin lesions with GANs; 2018. arXiv preprint 180901410
19. Wehbe RM, Sheng J, Dutta S, et al. An artificial intelligence algorithm to detect COVID-19 on chest radiographs trained and tested on a large U.S. Clinical data set. Radiology. 2021;299(1):E167–76
20. Tejedor M, Woldaregay A, Godtliebsen F. Reinforcement learning application in diabetes blood glucose control: a systematic review. Artif Intell Med. 2020;104:101836
21. Tseng H, Luo Y, Cui S, et al. Deep reinforcement learning for automated radiation adaptation in lung cancer. Med Phys. 2017;44(12):66906705
22. Petersen B, Yang J, Grathwohl W, et al. Precision medicine as a control problem: using simulation and deep reinforcement learning to discover adaptive, personalized multi-cytokine therapy for sepsis; 2018. Preprint. arXiv:1802.10440
23. Komorowski M, CeliL A, Badawi O, et al. The Artificial Intelligence Clinician learns optimal treatment strategies for sepsis in intensive care. Nat Med. 2018;24:1716–20
24. Spampinato C, Palazzo S, Giordano D, et al. Deep learning for automated skeletal bone age assessment in X-ray images. Medl Image Anal. 2017;36:41–51
25. Miotto R, Li L, Kidd B, et al. Deep patient: an unsupervised representation to predict the future of patients from the electronic health records. Sci Rep. 2016;6
26. Hannun AY, Rajpurkar P, Haghpanahi M, et al. Cardiologist-level arrhythmia detection and classification in ambulatory electrocardiograms using a deep neural network. Nat Med. 2019;25:65–9

27. Razavian N, Marcus J, Sontag D. Multi-task prediction of disease onsets from longitudinal lab tests; 2016. arXiv preprint 160800647v3
28. Tian T, Wan J, Song Q, et al. Clustering single-cell RNA-seq data with a model-based deep learning approach. Nat Mach Intell. 2019;1:191–8

Chapter 2
Mathematical Encoding of Medical Data

As we saw in Chap. 1, data is the single most important ingredient in developing effective machine learning models. Medical data come in a variety of shapes and formats, ranging from clinical images (pathology slides, computed tomography scans, magnetic resonance images, etc.) to electrical bio-signals (electrocardiograms, electroencephalograms, electromyograms, etc.), to text data (patient notes, diagnosis and medication records, etc.), to genetic data (data from genome-wide association studies, sequencing, and gene expression data, etc.), and more.

In this chapter, we study common types and modalities of medical data used in modern machine learning, with a special focus on data transformations that are required before raw input data can be fed into machine learning models. In the process of introducing these data types, we review rudimentary but important concepts from linear algebra that enable representation and manipulation of data using mathematical constructs such as vectors, matrices, and tensors.

Numerical Data

Consider the following toy dataset consisting of 5 patients' systolic blood pressure values measured (in millimeter of mercury or mmHG) at the time of admission to the hospital

$$\begin{aligned} &\text{patient 1: } 124, \\ &\text{patient 2: } 227, \\ &\text{patient 3: } 105, \\ &\text{patient 4: } 160, \\ &\text{patient 5: } 202. \end{aligned} \tag{2.1}$$

R. Borhani et al., *Fundamentals of Machine Learning and Deep Learning in Medicine*, https://doi.org/10.1007/978-3-031-19502-0_2

In mathematics, data like this is typically stored in, and represented by, an object called a *vector* that is simply an ordered listing of numbers

$$\mathbf{x} = [124 \quad 227 \quad 105 \quad 160 \quad 202]\,. \tag{2.2}$$

Throughout the book, we represent vectors by a bold lowercase (often Roman) letter such as $\mathbf{x}$ in order to distinguish them from scalar values that are typically denoted by non-bold Roman or Greek letters such as x or α.

When the *elements* or *entries* inside a vector are listed out horizontally (or in a row) as in (2.2), we call the resulting vector a *row vector*. Alternatively, the vector's entries can be listed vertically (or in a column), in which case we refer to the resulting vector as a *column* vector. We can always swap back and forth between the row and column versions of the vector via a vector operation called *transposition*. Notationally, transposition is denoted by the letter T placed just to the right and above a vector that turns a row vector into a column vector and vice versa, e.g.,

$$\mathbf{x}^T = [124 \quad 227 \quad 105 \quad 160 \quad 202]^T = \begin{bmatrix} 124 \\ 227 \\ 105 \\ 160 \\ 202 \end{bmatrix}. \tag{2.3}$$

In general, a vector can have an arbitrary number of elements, which is referred to as its *dimension*. For example, the vectors $\mathbf{x}$ and $\mathbf{y}$

$$\mathbf{x} = \begin{bmatrix} x_1 \\ x_2 \\ \vdots \\ x_N \end{bmatrix}, \quad \mathbf{y} = \begin{bmatrix} y_1 \\ y_2 \\ \vdots \\ y_N \end{bmatrix} \tag{2.4}$$

are both N-dimensional or of dimension N. Because $\mathbf{x}$ and $\mathbf{y}$ have the same dimension and orientation (i.e., they are both column vectors), we can add them together element-wise to form their addition that can be written as

$$\mathbf{x} + \mathbf{y} = \begin{bmatrix} x_1 + y_1 \\ x_2 + y_2 \\ \vdots \\ x_N + y_N \end{bmatrix}. \tag{2.5}$$

Subtraction of $\mathbf{y}$ from $\mathbf{x}$ can be defined similarly as

$$\mathbf{x} - \mathbf{y} = \begin{bmatrix} x_1 - y_1 \\ x_2 - y_2 \\ \vdots \\ x_N - y_N \end{bmatrix}. \tag{2.6}$$

Aside from the rudimentary operations of addition and subtraction, the two vectors **x** and **y** in (2.4) can also be multiplied together in a number of ways, one of which called the *inner-product* is of particular interest to us in this book. Also referred to as the *dot-product*, the inner-product of **x** and **y** produces a scalar output that is the sum of the pair-wise multiplication of the corresponding entries in **x** and **y**. Denoted by $\mathbf{x}^T\mathbf{y}$, the inner-product of **x** and **y** can be written as

$$\mathbf{x}^T\mathbf{y} = [x_1 \ x_2 \ \cdots \ x_N] \begin{bmatrix} y_1 \\ y_2 \\ \vdots \\ y_N \end{bmatrix} = x_1y_1 + x_2y_2 + \cdots + x_Ny_N = \sum_{n=1}^{N} x_ny_n. \tag{2.7}$$

When a vector **x** is multiplied by a scalar α, the resulting vector will have all its entries scaled by α

$$\alpha\,\mathbf{x} = \begin{bmatrix} \alpha\,x_1 \\ \alpha\,x_2 \\ \vdots \\ \alpha\,x_N \end{bmatrix}. \tag{2.8}$$

Because our senses have evolved in a world with three physical dimensions, we can understand one-, two-, and three-dimensional vectors intuitively. For instance, as illustrated in the left panel of Fig. 2.1, we can visualize two-dimensional vectors as arrows stemming from the origin in a two-dimensional plane. Addition of two vectors as well as vector–scalar multiplication is also easy to interpret geometrically as shown via examples in the middle and right panels of Fig. 2.1, respectively.

Thinking of vectors as arrows helps us define the *norm* (or magnitude) of a vector as the length of the arrow representing it. For a general two-dimensional vector

$$\mathbf{x} = \begin{bmatrix} x_1 \\ x_2 \end{bmatrix}, \tag{2.9}$$

the Pythagorean theorem provides a simple formula to calculate the norm of **x** denoted by the notation $\|\mathbf{x}\|$, as

$$\|\mathbf{x}\| = \sqrt{x_1^2 + x_2^2}, \tag{2.10}$$

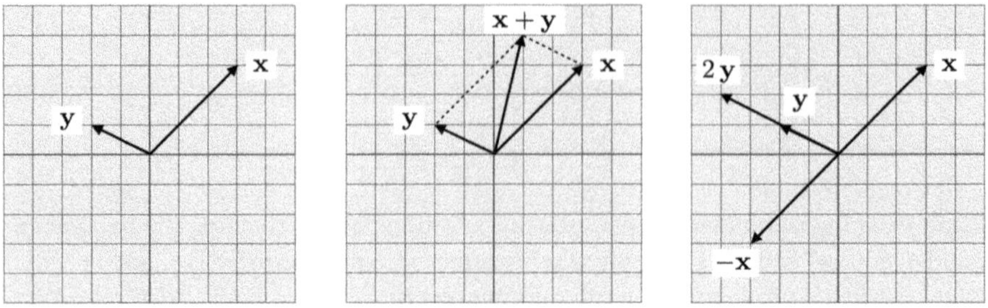

Fig. 2.1 (Left panel) Vectors $\mathbf{x} = [3 \;\; 3]$ and $\mathbf{y} = [-2 \;\; 1]$ drawn as arrows starting from the origin and ending at points whose horizontal and vertical coordinates are stored in $\mathbf{x}$ and $\mathbf{y}$, respectively. (middle panel) The addition of $\mathbf{x}$ and $\mathbf{y}$ is equal to the vector connecting the origin to the opposite corner of the parallelogram that has $\mathbf{x}$ and $\mathbf{y}$ as its sides. (right panel) When multiplied by a scalar α, the resulting vector will remain in parallel to the original vector, but its length will alter depending on the magnitude of α. Note that when α is negative, the resulting vector will point in the opposite direction of the original vector

which can be expressed equivalently as the square root of the inner-product of $\mathbf{x}$ and itself, or $\sqrt{\mathbf{x}^T\mathbf{x}}$. This also generalizes to vectors of any dimension meaning that when $\mathbf{x}$ is in general N-dimensional, we can similarly define its norm as[1]

$$\|\mathbf{x}\| = \sqrt{\mathbf{x}^T\mathbf{x}} = \sqrt{x_1^2 + x_2^2 + \cdots + x_N^2}. \tag{2.11}$$

So far we have pictured vectors as arrows stemming from the origin. This is the conventional way vectors are usually depicted in any standard mathematics or linear algebra text. However in the context of deep learning and as illustrated in Fig. 2.2, it is often more visually helpful to draw vectors not as a set of arrows but as a scattering of dots encoding the location of each arrow's endpoint or spike.

Categorical Data

Mathematical functions used in the context of deep learning require inputs that are strictly numerical or quantitative, as was the case with systolic blood pressure mentioned in the previous section. However, medical data does not always come prepackaged in this manner. Sometime medical variables of interest are *categorical* in nature. For instance, the type of COVID-19 vaccine an individual receives in the United States does not take on a numerical value, but instead belongs to one of the following categories: Moderna, Pfizer-BioNTech (or Pfizer for short), and Johnson

[1] It should be noted that (2.11) represents the most common but only one of many ways in which the norm of a vector can be defined.

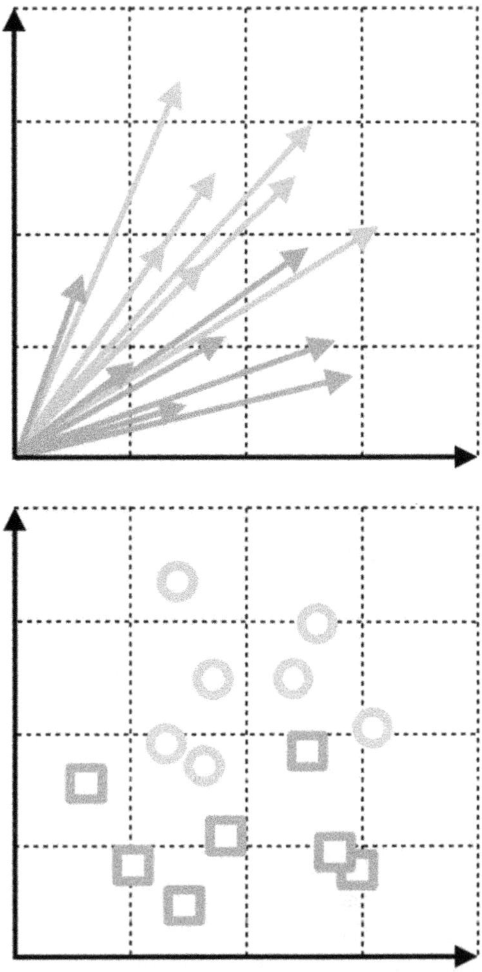

Fig. 2.2 The classification dataset shown originally in Fig. 1.10 from two different but equivalent perspectives: each instance of the data is represented as an arrow in the top panel and as a single point (square or circle) in the bottom panel. Clearly, the plot on the bottom is easier to visualize as a classification dataset than the one on the top

& Johnson's Janssen (or J&J for short). Such categories need to be translated into numerical values before they can be used by deep learning algorithms.

It is certainly possible to represent each category with a distinct number, for example, by assigning 1 to Moderna, 2 to Pfizer, and 3 to J&J. However as illustrated in the left panel of Fig. 2.3, by doing so, we have made the implicit assumption that the Pfizer vaccine (encoded with a value of 2) is closer or more "similar" to the J&J vaccine (encoded with a value of 3) than the Moderna vaccine (encoded with a value of 1). This assumption may or may not be true in reality. In general, it is best to avoid making such assumptions that could alter the problem's geometry, especially when we lack the intuition or knowledge necessary for ascertaining similarity or dissimilarity between different categories in the data.

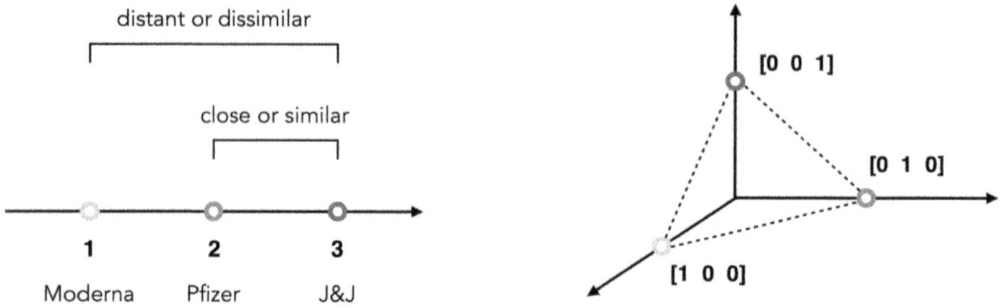

Fig. 2.3 Encoding of a categorical variable (i.e., the type of the COVID-19 vaccine administered in the United States) via a single number (left panel) and via one-hot encoding (right panel). See text for further details

One-hot encoding is the proper way to encode categorical variables in which each of the c categories is no longer represented by a single number, but instead by a vector of length c consisting of $c - 1$ "0"s and a single "1." This way the position of the only nonzero (hot) in the vector determines the identity of the category it encodes. In the case of the COVID-19 vaccine example discussed above, since there exist $c = 3$ categories in the data, we can represent the Moderna vaccine using the vector $[1\ 0\ 0]$, the Pfizer vaccine using $[0\ 1\ 0]$, and the J&J vaccine using $[0\ 0\ 1]$. Note that as shown in the right panel of Fig. 2.3, with one-hot encoding, the representations of all three categories are now geometrically equidistant from one another.

Imaging Data

Digital images are ubiquitous today and come in a wide variety of sizes, colors, and formats. We start with the most basic digital image, called a *black and white* or *binary* image, which can be represented as a two-dimensional array of bits (i.e., 0s and 1s) as illustrated in Fig. 2.4. Each cell in the array is called a *pixel* and is either black (if the pixel value is 0) or white (if the pixel value is 1).

In general, binary images are extremely limited in the amount of information they convey. This is because each pixel in a binary image can only hold one bit of information. To remedy, this limitation *grayscale* images allow every pixel to hold up to 8 bits (or 1 byte) of information. As a result, grayscale images can be composed of $2^8 = 256$ different shades of gray as illustrated in Fig. 2.5.

In addition to the number of bits used per pixel, the image *resolution* (i.e., the total number of pixels in the image) is also determinative of the amount of information held in an image. Intuitively, the higher the image resolution the more visual information can be stored in the image (see Fig. 2.6).

Given their two-dimensional nature, it is clear that we need mathematical objects other than vectors to store grayscale images. *Matrices* happen to be the ideal data

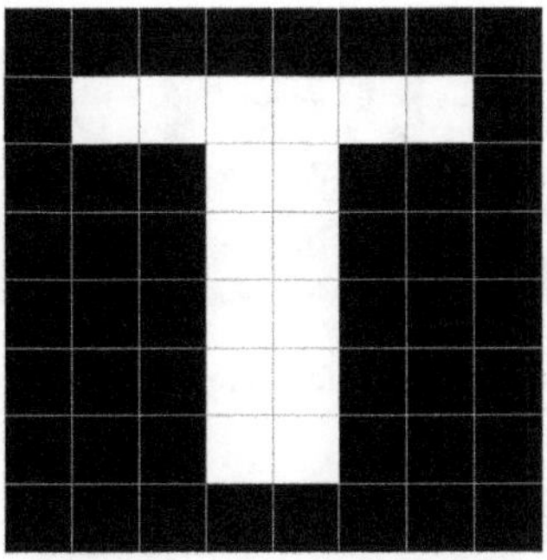

0	0	0	0	0	0	0	0
0	1	1	1	1	1	1	0
0	0	0	1	1	0	0	0
0	0	0	1	1	0	0	0
0	0	0	1	1	0	0	0
0	0	0	1	1	0	0	0
0	0	0	1	1	0	0	0
0	0	0	0	0	0	0	0

Fig. 2.4 A black and white image of the letter "T." Conventionally, black and white colors are assigned the values of 0 and 1, respectively

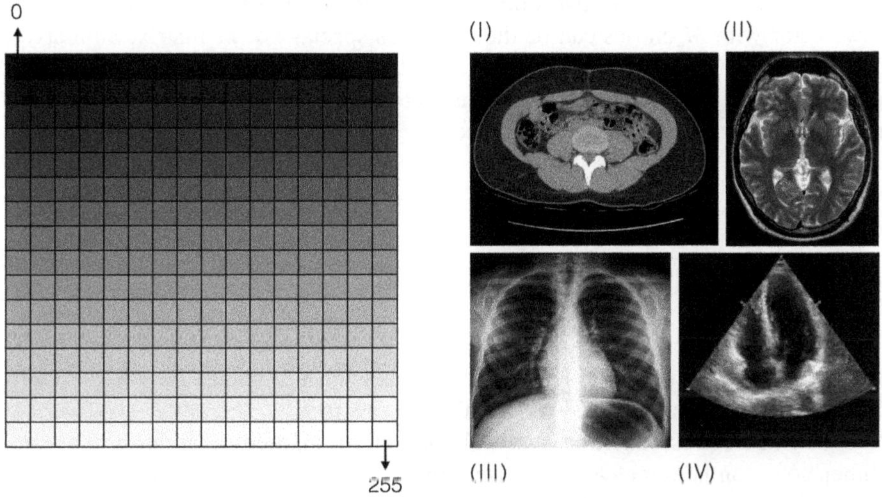

Fig. 2.5 (Left panel) Grayscale images are composed of 256 shades of gray, wherein each pixel takes an integer value in the range of 0 to 255, with 0 representing the smallest light intensity (black) and 255 representing the largest intensity (white). (Right panel) (I) CT-scans, (II) MRIs, (III) X-rays, (IV) echocardiograms, and many other imaging modalities used in modern medicine are grayscale images

structure for this purpose. An $N \times M$ matrix, denoted in this book by a bold uppercase letter such as **X**, is a two-dimensional array of numbers

$$\mathbf{X} = \begin{bmatrix} x_{11} & x_{12} & \cdots & x_{1M} \\ x_{21} & x_{22} & \cdots & x_{2M} \\ \vdots & \vdots & \ddots & \vdots \\ x_{N1} & x_{N2} & \cdots & x_{NM}, \end{bmatrix} \tag{2.12}$$

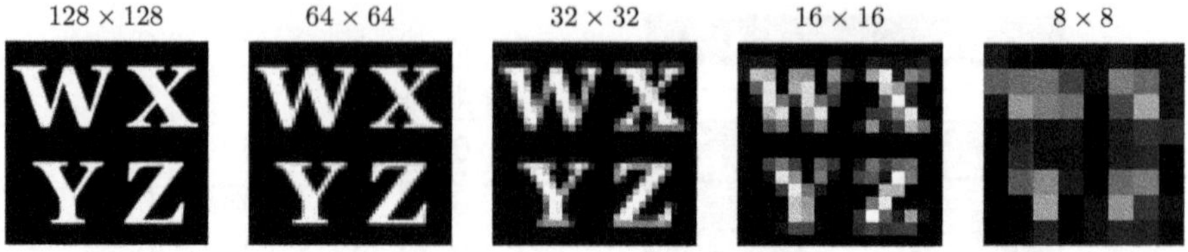

Fig. 2.6 Grayscale image of four alphabet letters visualized at different resolutions

which can be constructed either as a collection of N row vectors stacked on top of each other or as a collection of M column vectors stacked next to each other. For this reason, $\mathbf{X}$ is said to have N rows and M columns, with the entry in its ith row and jth column denoted as either $\mathbf{X}_{i,j}$ or more simply x_{ij}.

Matrices are essentially two-dimensional generalizations of vectors. As such, a row vector with M entries can be thought of as special $1 \times M$ matrix. Similarly, a column vector with N entries is an $N \times 1$ matrix. Many vector operations discussed previously in Sect. "Numerical Data" have corresponding analogs for matrices. For example, the transposition of $\mathbf{X}$, denoted as

$$\mathbf{X}^T = \begin{bmatrix} x_{11} & x_{21} & \cdots & x_{N1} \\ x_{12} & x_{22} & \cdots & x_{N2} \\ \vdots & \vdots & \ddots & \vdots \\ x_{1M} & x_{2M} & \cdots & x_{NM} \end{bmatrix}, \tag{2.13}$$

flips the whole matrix around so that the ith row in $\mathbf{X}$ becomes the ith column in $\mathbf{X}^T$, and the jth column in $\mathbf{X}$ becomes the jth row in $\mathbf{X}^T$.

As with vectors, addition and subtraction of matrices that have the same dimensions can be done element-wise, mirroring Equations (2.5) and (2.6). While the inner-product (or dot-product) is not defined for matrices, a common form of matrix multiplication is built upon the inner-product concept. To be able to multiply matrices $\mathbf{X}$ and $\mathbf{Y}$, the number of columns in the first matrix must match the number of rows in the second matrix. Assuming $\mathbf{X}$ and $\mathbf{Y}$ are $M \times N$ and $N \times P$, respectively, the product of $\mathbf{X}$ and $\mathbf{Y}$ (denoted as $\mathbf{XY}$) will be an $M \times P$ matrix whose (i, j)th entry is the inner-product of the ith row of $\mathbf{X}$ and the jth column of $\mathbf{Y}$. A simple example of matrix multiplication is shown in (2.14).

$$\begin{bmatrix} a & b \\ c & d \\ e & f \end{bmatrix} \begin{bmatrix} u & v & w \\ x & y & z \end{bmatrix} = \begin{bmatrix} au+bx & av+by & aw+bz \\ cu+dx & cv+dy & cw+dz \\ eu+fx & ev+fy & ew+fz \end{bmatrix}. \tag{2.14}$$

Just as with vectors, we can also define the norm of a matrix as a number representing its overall size. Recall from (2.11) that the norm of a vector is defined as the square root of the sum of the squares of its entries. The matrix norm is defined similarly as the square root of the sum of the squares of all the matrix entries, which can be written for the matrix $\mathbf{X}$ in (2.12) as[2]

$$\|\mathbf{X}\| = \sqrt{\sum_{n=1}^{N}\sum_{m=1}^{M} x_{nm}^2}. \tag{2.15}$$

As illustrated in Fig. 2.7, several medical imaging modalities produce color images that are different from grayscale images in terms of appearance and structure. Examples of color images used in the clinic include dermoscopy, ophthalmoscopy, cystoscopy, and colonoscopy images, to just name a few. A common way to create the perception of color is through superimposing the primary colors of red, green, and blue. In this color system, often referred to as the RGB system, the level or intensity of each of the three primary colors determines the final color resulted from their combination. Using the RGB system and assuming 256 levels of intensity for each of the primary colors, we can define $256 \times 256 \times 256 = 16,777,216$ unique colors, each represented by a triple in the form of $[r \ b \ g]$, where $0 \leq r, b, g \leq 255$ are integers (see the left panel of Fig. 2.7).

Since pixel values in an RGB image are no longer scalars, the matrix data structure shown in (2.12) is inadequate to support color images. To store such images, we need a new data structure called a *tensor* that is the natural extension of the two-dimensional matrix to three dimensions, just as the matrix itself was the

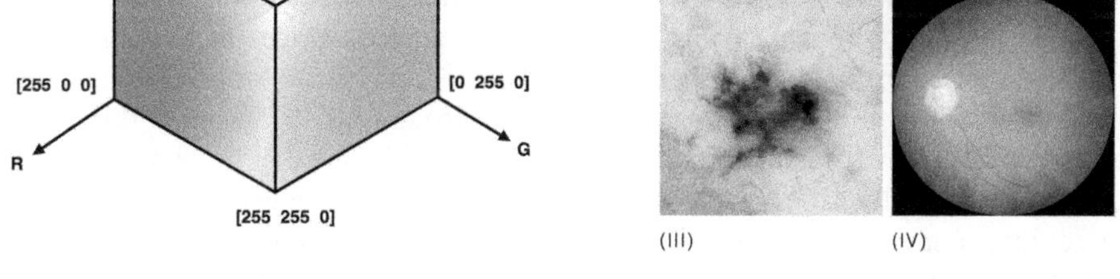

Fig. 2.7 (Left panel) The RGB color space. Each color in this space is represented as a triple of integers $[r \ b \ g]$ where $0 \leq r, b, g \leq 255$. (Right panel) (I) Colonoscopy images, (II) histology slides, (III) dermoscopy images, and (IV) ophthalmoscopy images are all examples of color imaging modalities

[2] The matrix norm defined in (2.15), often referred to as the Frobenius norm, is the most common but only one of many ways in which the norm of a matrix may be defined.

natural extension of vectors to two dimensions. An $M \times N \times P$ tensor is a three-dimensional structure with M rows, N columns, and P layers. We can therefore represent any RGB image using a tensor with $P = 3$ layers, one for each primary color.

Note that if needed, nothing stops us from extending the concept of a tensor to dimensions higher than three. In general, a rank-t tensor is an array whose every entry is a scalar that can be indexed by a t-dimensional vector. Using this overarching definition, vectors and matrices can be thought of as rank-1 and rank-2 tensors, respectively.

Time-Series Data

A time-series is a series or sequence of numerical values collected over time. In its most general form, a time-series can be represented as a sequence of time–value pairs

$$(t_1, x_1), (t_2, x_2), \ldots, (t_N, x_N), \tag{2.16}$$

where $t_1, t_2, \ldots, t_N$ are time-marks or time-stamps sorted in ascending order ($t_1 < t_2 < \cdots < t_N$), and $x_1, x_2, \ldots, x_N$ are the corresponding values of the quantity of interest captured at each time-mark. In the top-left panel of Fig. 2.8, we show a toy time-series dataset with $N = 5$ time–value pairs. In the top-right panel, we show the same dataset; only this time every two consecutive time–value pairs, i.e., (t_i, x_i) and (t_{i+1}, x_{i+1}), are connected via a line segment. Note that while these line segments are not part of the original data, their addition gives the data a more continuous appearance. The practice of connecting consecutive time–value pairs with a straight line segment is often referred to as linear interpolation and is done primarily to facilitate the visualization of such data.

In most circumstances, time-series data is collected at equally spaced points in time. In the bottom panel of Fig. 2.8, we show the stock prices of two American movie distribution companies (namely, Blockbuster and Netflix) reported on a daily basis over a period of seven years from 2003 through 2010. The time difference between any two consecutive data points in this case is one day or 24 h. This time difference, typically referred to the *temporal resolution*, can in general be smaller or larger than a day. For example, stock exchanges around the world now publish their data every few minutes, whereas the federal spending as a percentage of GDP in the United States, again a time-series data, is published only once a year.

Notice, when time-series data is captured at equally spaced points in time, we can conveniently drop the time-stamps $t_1, t_2, \ldots, t_N$ and represent the data in (2.16) more compactly as

$$x_1, x_2, \ldots, x_N. \tag{2.17}$$

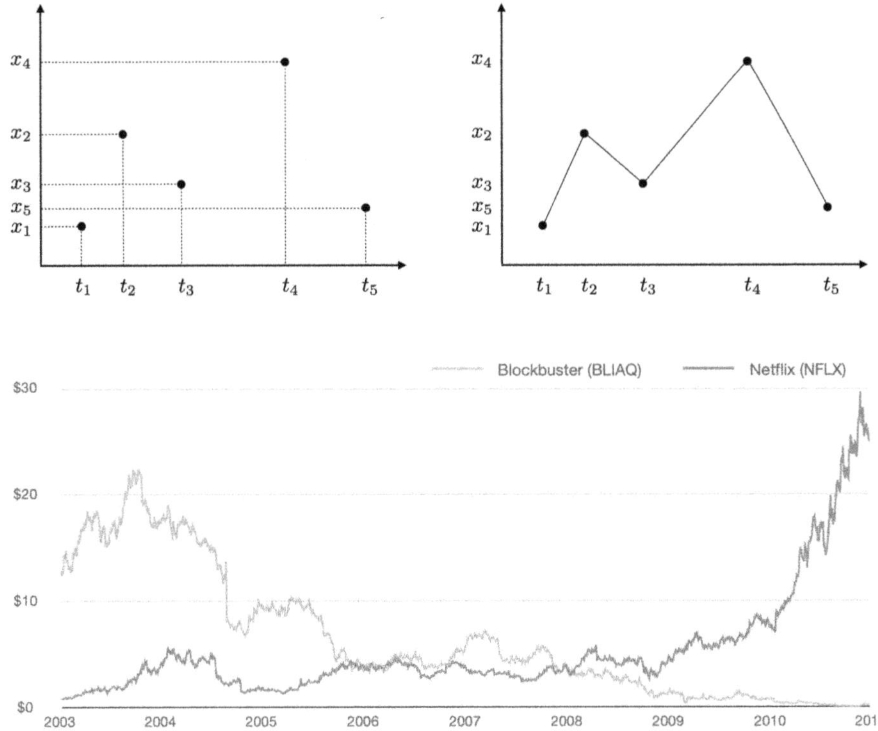

Fig. 2.8 (Top left panel) A toy time series dataset with $N = 5$ time–value pairs. (Top-right panel) Linear interpolation of the same dataset, done by connecting consecutive points with a line, makes it easier for the human eye to follow the ebb and flow in the data. (Bottom panel) Daily stock prices are a common instance of time-series data. Here, the daily stock prices of two movie distribution companies are plotted over a seven-year period from 2003 through 2010

As long as the initial time-stamp (t_1) and the temporal resolution ($t_2 - t_1$) are known, we can always use the compact representation above to revert back to the fuller representation in (2.16) if needed.

The most common time-series data encountered in medicine are electrical bio-signals such as electrocardiograms and electroencephalograms, as well as data generated from wearable technologies that can track different physical aspects of an individual's daily routine and movement over time.

An electrocardiogram (ECG) is inherently a time-series where the quantity measured over time is the electrical activity of the heart that conveys valuable information about the heart's structure and function. In the most conventional form of ECG, 10 electrodes are placed over different parts of the body as depicted in the top panel of Fig. 2.9. These electrodes, six placed over the chest and four on the limbs, measure small voltage changes induced throughout the body during each heartbeat. In the bottom panel of Fig. 2.9, we show the prototypical output of one of these electrodes in a healthy individual. Each unit in the horizontal direction (i.e.,

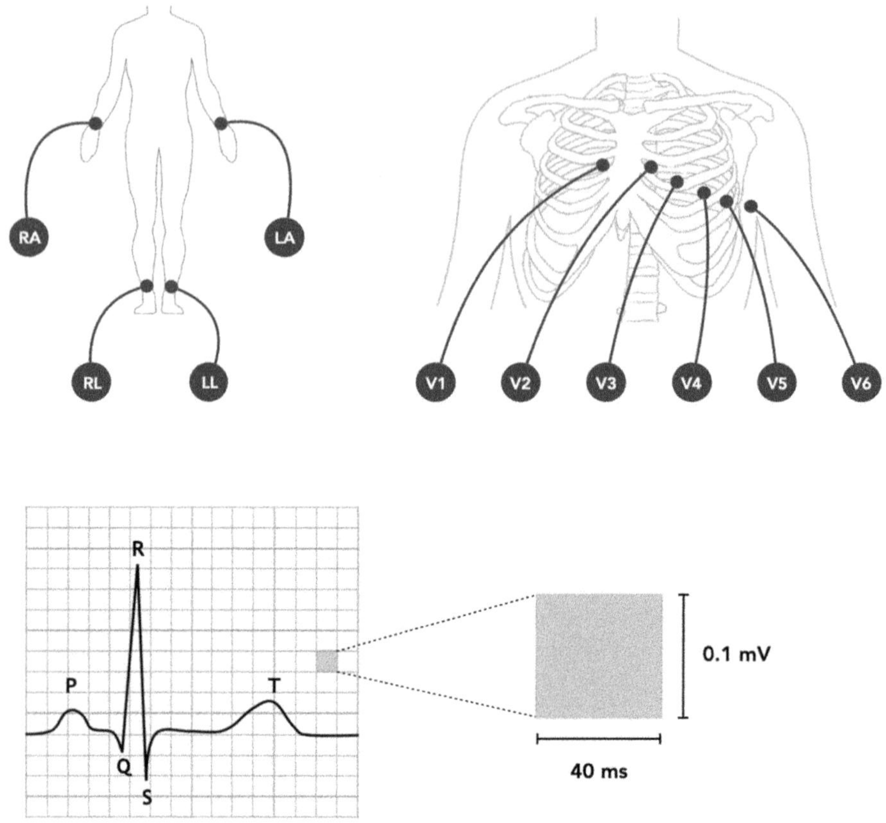

Fig. 2.9 (Top panel) The approximate position of the ECG electrodes on the body. (Bottom panel) The graph of voltage versus time for one cardiac cycle (heartbeat)

time) represents 40 milliseconds (ms), whereas each unit in the vertical direction (i.e., voltage) represents 0.1 millivolts (mV). As can be seen in the figure, the voltage pattern associated with a normal heartbeat consists of three distinct components: the P wave, the QRS complex, and the T wave, each representing the changes in electrical activity of the heart muscle that happen as a result of contraction and relaxation of its chambers. Deviations from the normal P-QRS-T patterns can be used as a basis to diagnose a host of medical conditions including myocardial ischemia/infarction, arrhythmias, myocardial hypertrophy, myocarditis, pericarditis, pericardial effusion, valvular diseases, and certain electrolyte imbalances, to name a few.

The readings from three of the limb electrodes shown in Fig. 2.9 (namely, RA, LA, and LL) are linearly combined to produce six *lead* signals (namely, I, II, III, aVR, aVL, and aVF) defined, respectively, as

$$\begin{aligned}
\text{I} &= \text{LA} - \text{RA}, \\
\text{II} &= \text{LL} - \text{RA}, \\
\text{III} &= \text{LL} - \text{LA}, \\
\text{aVR} &= \text{RA} - \frac{\text{LA} + \text{LL}}{2}, \\
\text{aVL} &= \text{LA} - \frac{\text{RA} + \text{LL}}{2}, \\
\text{aVF} &= \text{LL} - \frac{\text{RA} + \text{LA}}{2}.
\end{aligned} \tag{2.18}$$

Using vector and matrix notation, we can write the system of equations in (2.18) more compactly as

$$\begin{bmatrix} \text{I} \\ \text{II} \\ \text{III} \\ \text{aVR} \\ \text{aVL} \\ \text{aVF} \end{bmatrix} = \begin{bmatrix} -1 & 1 & 0 \\ -1 & 0 & 1 \\ 0 & -1 & 1 \\ 1 & -0.5 & -0.5 \\ -0.5 & 1 & -0.5 \\ -0.5 & -0.5 & 1 \end{bmatrix} \begin{bmatrix} \text{RA} \\ \text{LA} \\ \text{LL} \end{bmatrix}. \tag{2.19}$$

The six lead signals defined in (2.19) are usually stitched together along with an additional set of lead signals read directly from the six chest electrodes to produce a so-called 12 lead ECG, an instance of which is shown in Fig. 2.10.

Text Data

In the context of medicine, textual information is generated routinely (and in large quantities) in the form of electronic health records (EHRs) comprising patient notes, physical evaluation and examination records, medication orders, radiology and pathology reports, discharge summaries, etc. One important aspect in which text data is different from other data types we have discussed so far is that it is usually generated by humans (e.g., doctors, nurses, healthcare workers, etc.) as opposed to other data types that are typically generated by machines (e.g., imaging scanners, ECG monitors, etc.). As a result of this distinction in the source of the data, there is naturally more inherent variability in the former compared to the latter group.

To better highlight this point, consider the hypothetical example of a patient who visits two different dermatologists to assess a newly formed mole on his forearm. Both dermatologists take an image of the mole and provide a written description of its appearance (see Fig. 2.11). Notice, while the two images are not identical (since they were acquired using different cameras, from different angles,

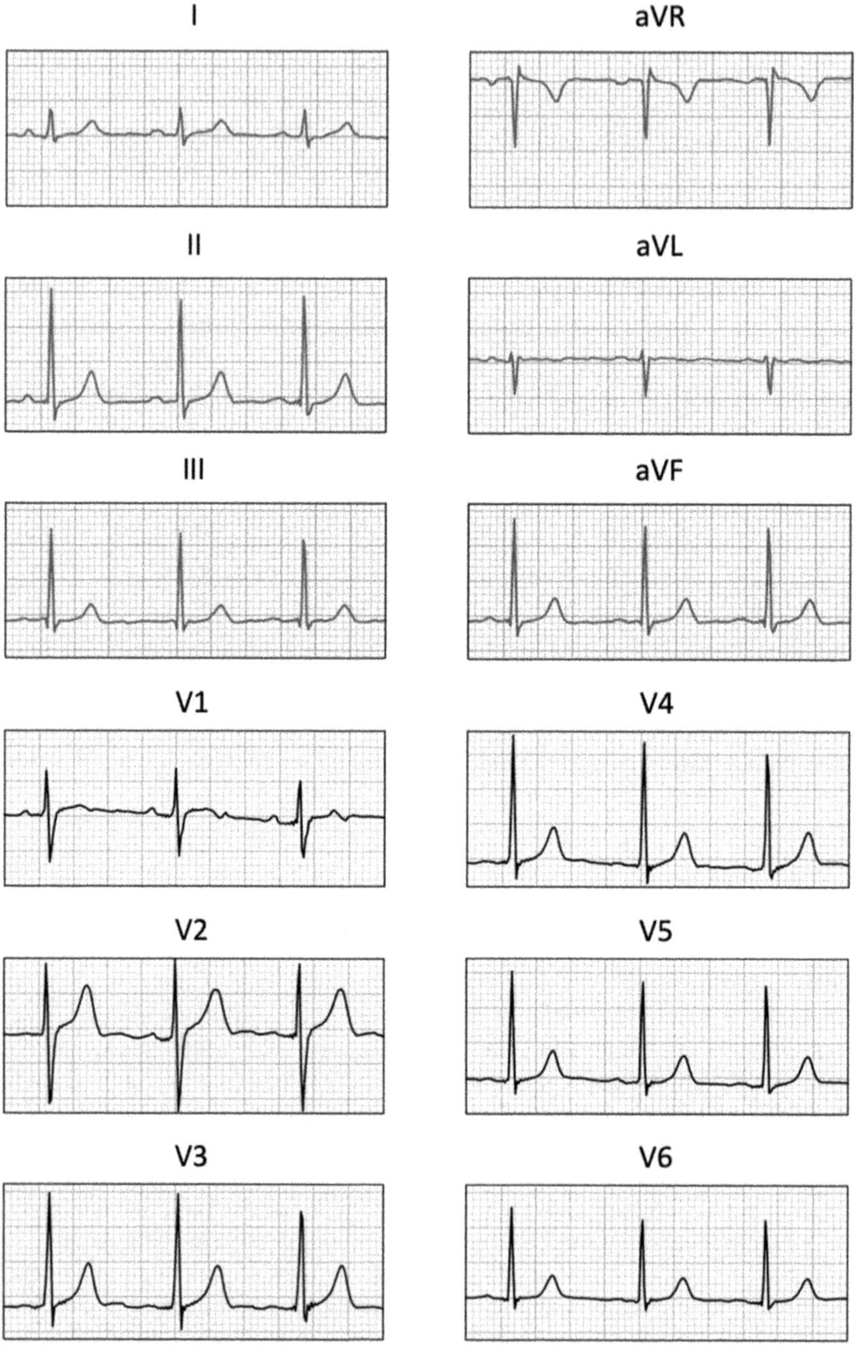

Fig. 2.10 A 12 lead ECG is a collection of six lead signals from the chest and six lead signals from the limbs as defined in (2.19)

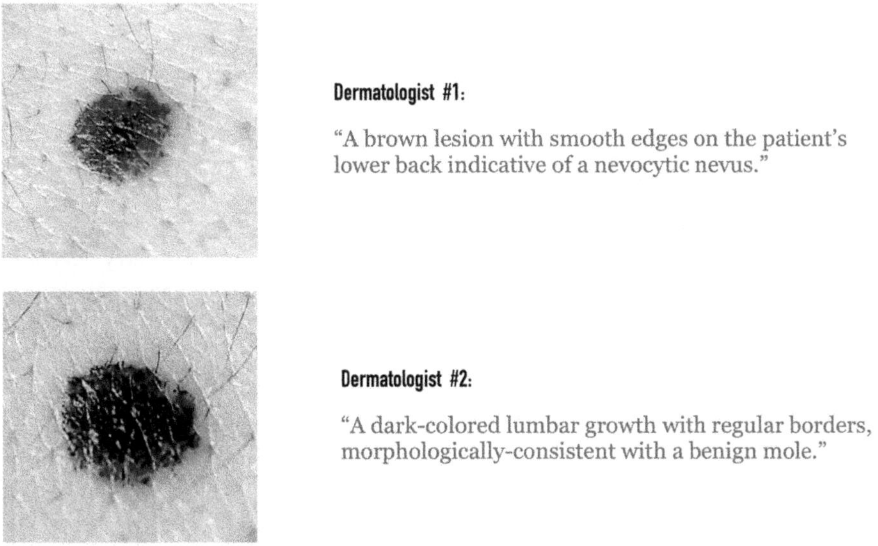

Fig. 2.11 Generally speaking, human-generated data (here, written descriptions of a mole by two dermatologists) have more intrinsic variability than machine-generated data (here, dermoscopy images of the same mole). See text for further details

and under different lighting conditions), they are much more alike compared to their corresponding written descriptions. Because humans can express the same idea or sentiment in a multitude of ways, the processing of natural languages (e.g., written text) can be considerably more challenging than that of natural signals (e.g., images). Hence, when it comes to text documents and files, the raw input data usually requires a significant amount of preprocessing, normalization, and transformation.

A *bag of words* (or BoW for short) is a simple, commonly used, vector-based normalization and transformation scheme for text documents. In its most basic form, a BoW vector representation consists of the normalized count of different words used in a text document with respect to a single corpus or a collection of documents, excluding those non-distinctive words that do not characterize the document in the context of the application at hand.

To illustrate this idea, in what follows, we build a BoW representation for a toy text dataset in (2.22) comprising two *progress notes* that describe the patients' clinical status during their stay in the hospital.

1. "Patient was sent to the ICU because of respiratory failure."
2. "Patient's fever, respiratory rate, and respiratory alkalosis have improved."

(2.20)

To create the BoW representation of these two single-sentence text documents, we first remove spaces and punctuation marks, along with other uninformative words

alkalosis	because	fail	fever	ICU	improve	patient	rate	respirate	send
0	1	1	0	1	0	1	0	1	1
1	0	0	1	0	1	1	1	2	0

Fig. 2.12 Bag of words (BoW) representation of the two text documents shown in (2.22). See text for details

such as `and`, `have`, `of`, `the`, `to`, and `was`. These words, typically referred to as *stop words*, are so commonly used in the English language that they carry very little useful information and hence can be removed without severely compromising the document's syntax. Additionally, we can reduce each remaining word to its stem or root form. For example, since the words `improve`, `improved`, `improving`, `improvement`, and `improvements` all have the same common linguistic root, we can represent them all using the word `improve` without too much information loss. These preprocessing steps transform the original dataset displayed in (2.22) into the one shown in (2.21).

1. `patient`, `send`, `ICU`, `because`, `respirate`, `fail`
2. `patient`, `fever`, `respirate`, `rate`, `respirate`, `alkalosis`, `improve`

(2.21)

Next, for each document, we form a vector containing the number of times each word appears in it. As illustrated in Fig. 2.12, the dimension of this vector is equal to the total number of unique words used across our dataset (here, 10). Finally, it is common practice to divide each BoW vector by its norm so that all resulting BoW vectors have unit length.

Note that because the BoW representation only captures the number of times each word appears in a text document and *not* its location within the document, it can only provide a gross summary of the document's contents. While this per se does not rule out the use of the bag of words scheme in many text-based applications, one should be cognizant of this weakness before employing this scheme in practice. For instance, using BoW representation, the two following statements

1. "Paracetamol is more effective than Ibuprofen in these patients."
2. "Ibuprofen is more effective than Paracetamol in these patients."

(2.22)

would be considered identical even though they imply completely opposite meanings. To remedy this problem, another popular text encoding scheme treats documents like a time-series. Recall from Sect. "Time-Series Data" that time-series data (when the time increments are all equal) can be represented as an ordered listing or a sequence of *numbers*. Text data can similarly be thought of as a sequence of *characters* made up of letters, numbers, spaces, and other special characters (e.g., "%," "!," "@," etc.). In Table 2.1, we show a subset of alphanumeric characters along with their ASCII codes. An abbreviation for the American Standard Code for Information Interchange, ASCII, is a universal character-encoding standard for electronic communications in which every character is assigned a numerical code that can be stored in computer memory. For instance, a medication order that reads

$$\texttt{GIVE 1 MG QID,} \tag{2.23}$$

which instructs the patient be given one milligram of a certain drug four times a day, can be stored in the computer using the following ASCII representation:

$$[71,\ 73,\ 86,\ 69,\ 32,\ 49,\ 32,\ 77,\ 71,\ 32,\ 81,\ 73,\ 68]. \tag{2.24}$$

Note, however, that this representation still suffers from the same sort of problem described in Sect. "Categorical Data" and visualized in Fig. 2.3. That is, since alphanumeric characters are *categorical* in nature, representing them using numbers (e.g., ASCII codes) is sub-optimal for deep learning purposes. Instead, it is best to employ an encoding scheme such as *one-hot encoding*, replacing each ASCII entry in (2.24) with its corresponding one-hot encoded vector from Table 2.1. Finally, it should be noted that while the representation shown in (2.24) was based on a *character-level* parsing of the text in (2.23), similar representations can be constructed at the *word level* as well.

Genomics Data

The genetic information required for the biological functioning and reproduction of all living organisms is contained within an organic compound called deoxyribonucleic acid or DNA for short. The DNA molecule is a long chain of repeating chemical units or bases strung together in the shape of two twisting strands, as illustrated in Fig. 2.13. Each strand is made of four bases: adenine, cytosine, guanine, and thymine, which are commonly abbreviated as `A`, `C`, `G`, and `T`, respectively.

Structurally, adenine bases in one strand always face thymine bases in the opposite strand and vice versa. Similarly, cytosine bases in one strand always pair with thymine bases in the other and vice versa. Because of this redundancy, the entire DNA structure can be fully characterized using only one of its strands.
From a data structure perspective, the DNA molecule is a very long[3] piece of text written in a language whose alphabet consists of four letters only. We can therefore treat DNA sequences as text data and apply the transformations discussed previously in Sect. "Text Data". For example, the length-9 sequence

$$\texttt{A A C T G T C A G} \tag{2.25}$$

can be represented using a one-hot encoding scheme, as the 4×9 matrix

[3] The human DNA is estimated to be composed of more than three billion bases!

Table 2.1 ASCII and one-hot encoded representations of the space character, single-digit numbers, and uppercase letters of the alphabet

Character	ASCII Code	One-hot encoded vector
	32	[1000000000000000000000000000000000000]
0	48	[0100000000000000000000000000000000000]
1	49	[0010000000000000000000000000000000000]
2	50	[0001000000000000000000000000000000000]
3	51	[0000100000000000000000000000000000000]
4	52	[0000010000000000000000000000000000000]
5	53	[0000001000000000000000000000000000000]
6	54	[0000000100000000000000000000000000000]
7	55	[0000000010000000000000000000000000000]
8	56	[0000000001000000000000000000000000000]
9	57	[0000000000100000000000000000000000000]
A	65	[0000000000010000000000000000000000000]
B	66	[0000000000001000000000000000000000000]
C	67	[0000000000000100000000000000000000000]
D	68	[0000000000000010000000000000000000000]
E	69	[0000000000000001000000000000000000000]
F	70	[0000000000000000100000000000000000000]
G	71	[0000000000000000010000000000000000000]
H	72	[0000000000000000001000000000000000000]
I	73	[0000000000000000000100000000000000000]
J	74	[0000000000000000000010000000000000000]
K	75	[0000000000000000000001000000000000000]
L	76	[0000000000000000000000100000000000000]
M	77	[0000000000000000000000010000000000000]
N	78	[0000000000000000000000001000000000000]
O	79	[0000000000000000000000000100000000000]
P	80	[0000000000000000000000000010000000000]
Q	81	[0000000000000000000000000001000000000]
R	82	[0000000000000000000000000000100000000]
S	83	[0000000000000000000000000000010000000]
T	84	[0000000000000000000000000000001000000]
U	86	[0000000000000000000000000000000100000]
V	87	[0000000000000000000000000000000010000]
W	88	[0000000000000000000000000000000001000]
X	89	[0000000000000000000000000000000000100]
Y	90	[0000000000000000000000000000000000010]
Z	91	[0000000000000000000000000000000000001]

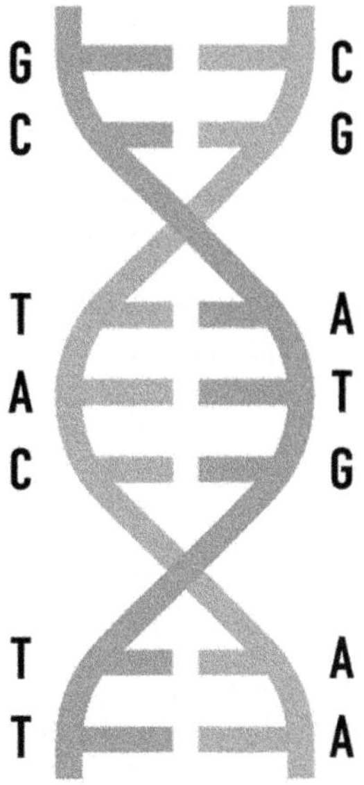

Fig. 2.13 The DNA molecule consists of two complementary chains twisting around one another to form a double helix. Every adenine (A) base in one chain faces a thymine (T) base in the other chain, and every cytosine (C) base in one chain is paired with a guanine (G) base in the other

$$\begin{bmatrix} 1\,1\,0\,0\,0\,0\,0\,1\,0 \\ 0\,0\,1\,0\,0\,0\,1\,0\,0 \\ 0\,0\,0\,0\,1\,0\,0\,0\,1 \\ 0\,0\,0\,1\,0\,1\,0\,0\,0 \end{bmatrix}, \tag{2.26}$$

where each column is a one-hot encoded vector representing one of the four bases in (2.25).

Another commonly used modality of genomics data are gene expression microarrays discussed briefly in Sect. "The Machine Learning Taxonomy". Unlike traditional low-throughput lab techniques such as real-time polymerase chain reaction (qPCR) and northern blot that can only handle a small number of genes per study, the microarray technology allows for simultaneous measurement of the expression levels of thousands of genes across an arbitrarily large population of patients. From a data structure point of view, this type of data can be stored in a matrix whose rows and columns represent patients and genes, respectively. The (i, j)th entry of the said matrix is a real number representing the expression level of gene j in patient i. This technology has been successfully applied to discovering novel disease subtypes (see Fig. 1.16) and identifying the underlying mechanisms of response to drugs.

Problems

2.1 Data Type and Dimension

Determine the proper type and dimension of the data structure needed to represent each of the following medical data objects:

(a) Demographic information including age, sex, and race for a cohort of patients
(b) A black and white picture of an ECG printout
(c) A high-resolution pathology slide of breast tissue suspected of malignancy
(d) A volumetric CT of the lung
(e) A functional magnetic resonance image (fMRI) that measures the activity in every volumetric pixel (or voxel) of the brain over a relatively short time window

2.2 Vector Calculations
Supposing

$$\mathbf{x} = \begin{bmatrix} -1 \\ 1 \\ 0 \end{bmatrix}, \quad \mathbf{y} = \begin{bmatrix} 2 \\ 5 \\ -1 \end{bmatrix}, \quad \text{and} \quad \mathbf{z} = \begin{bmatrix} 0 \\ 0 \\ -3 \end{bmatrix}, \tag{2.27}$$

compute the result of each of the following expressions:

(a) $\mathbf{x} + \mathbf{y} + \mathbf{z}$.
(b) $\mathbf{x}^T\mathbf{y} + \mathbf{y}^T\mathbf{z} + \mathbf{z}^T\mathbf{x}$.
(c) $\|\mathbf{x} + \mathbf{y} + \mathbf{z}\|$.
(d) $\|\mathbf{x}\| + \|\mathbf{y}\| + \|\mathbf{z}\|$.

2.3 Geometry of Vector Inner-Products

(a) Use the definition in (2.7) to find the inner-product of the vector $\mathbf{x}$ and each of the eight vectors $\mathbf{y}_1$ through $\mathbf{y}_8$ shown in Fig. 2.14.
(b) For each pair of vectors $(\mathbf{x}, \mathbf{y}_i)$ in part (a) find the corresponding vector norms $\|\mathbf{x}\|$ and $\|\mathbf{y}_i\|$, as well as the angle θ_i between $\mathbf{x}$ and $\mathbf{y}_i$, and confirm that the inner-product of $\mathbf{x}$ and $\mathbf{y}_i$ is equal to $\|\mathbf{x}\| \, \|\mathbf{y}_i\| \cos(\theta_i)$ for all $i = 1, 2, \ldots, 8$.
(c) The identity $\mathbf{x}^T\mathbf{y} = \|\mathbf{x}\| \, \|\mathbf{y}\| \cos(\theta)$ is true in general for any pair of vectors $\mathbf{x}$ and $\mathbf{y}$ of the same dimension. Use this rule to prove that the inner-product of two nonzero vectors is zero if and only if the two vectors are *perpendicular* or *orthogonal* to each other.

2.4 Properties of Vector Norms
Use the definition in (2.11) to:

(a) Show that the norm of any vector $\mathbf{x}$ is always non-negative. More precisely, prove that $\|\mathbf{x}\| \geq 0$ and the equality holds if and only if $\mathbf{x}$ has no other entry besides zero.
(b) Express $\|\alpha\mathbf{x}\|$ in terms of $\|\mathbf{x}\|$ and α, where α is a scalar (real number).
(c) Show that for all vectors $\mathbf{x}$ and $\mathbf{y}$ of the same dimension, we can always write $\|\mathbf{x}\| + \|\mathbf{y}\| \geq \|\mathbf{x} + \mathbf{y}\|$. In proving this inequality, commonly referred to as the *triangle inequality*, you may find it useful to employ the inner-product rule in part (c) of Exercise 2.3.

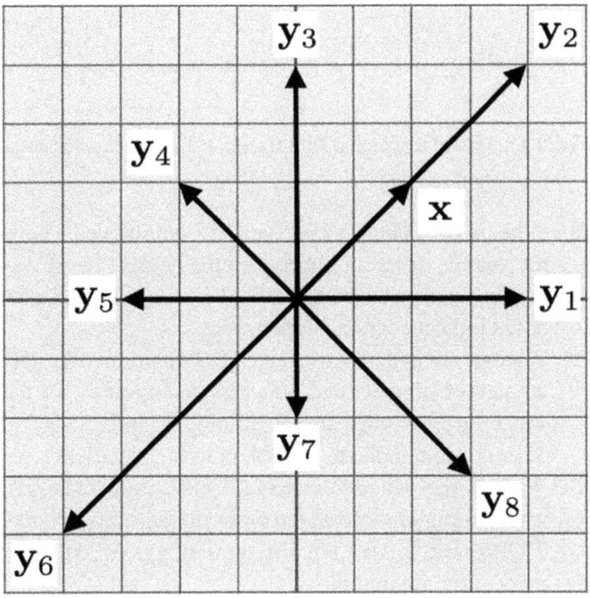

Fig. 2.14 Figure associated with Exercise 2.3. See text for details

2.5 Matrix Calculations

Supposing

$$\mathbf{A} = \begin{bmatrix} 1 & 1 \\ -1 & 2 \\ 0 & -1 \end{bmatrix}, \quad \mathbf{B} = \begin{bmatrix} 2 & 0 \\ -1 & 1 \end{bmatrix}, \quad \text{and} \quad \mathbf{x} = \begin{bmatrix} 1 \\ -1 \end{bmatrix}, \tag{2.28}$$

compute the result of each of the following expressions:

(a) $\mathbf{Ax}$.
(b) $\mathbf{x}^T\mathbf{Bx}$.
(c) $\|\mathbf{A}\| \times \|\mathbf{B}\|$.
(d) $\|\mathbf{AB}\|$.

2.6 One-Hot Encoding

Use Table 2.1 to determine the one-hot encoded representation of the medication order shown originally in (2.23).

2.7 ECG Calculations

Figure 2.15 shows multiple cardiac cycles of a certain lead of ECG in an adult patient. Use the information provided in Sect. "Time-Series Data" to answer the following questions:

(a) What is the patient's heart rate? Express your answer in terms of the number of beats per minute (bpm). A heart rate of less than 60 bpm indicates bradycardia.

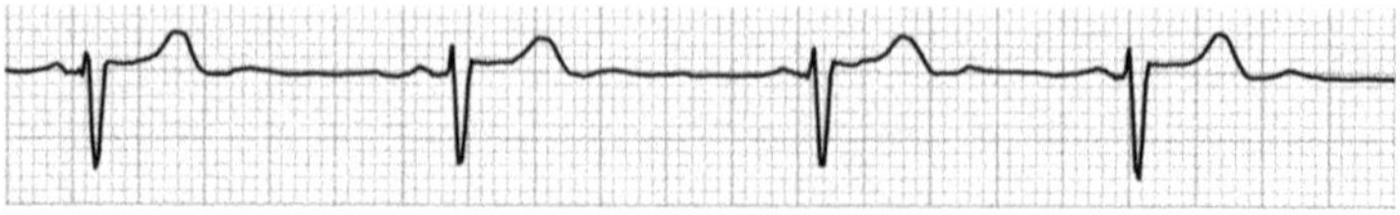

Fig. 2.15 Figure associated with Exercise 2.7. See text for details

(b) What is the patient's average QRS amplitude? The QRS amplitude is measured as the voltage differential between the peak of the R wave and the peak of the S wave. Express your answer in millivolts (mV). A QRS amplitude of greater than 4.5 mV could indicate cardiac hypertrophy.

(c) What is the patient's average QRS duration? The QRS duration is measured as the amount of time elapsed between the beginning of the Q wave and the end of the S wave. Express your answer in milliseconds (ms). A QRS duration of greater than 120 ms could indicate a problem in the electrical conduction system of the heart.

(d) What is the patient's average T/QRS ratio? The T/QRS ratio is defined as the T wave amplitude (measured from the baseline) divided by the QRS amplitude. The T/QRS ratio is useful in differentiating between left ventricular aneurysm and acute myocardial infarction.

Chapter 3
Elementary Functions and Operations

Having introduced data as a building block of machine learning systems in the previous chapter, here we discuss the basics of another vitally important building block: the mathematical function. In science and medicine, mathematical functions are so ubiquitous that most readers have certainly encountered them in some fashion at some point in their lives. In machine learning in particular, we are always dealing with mathematical functions: from the framing of a learning problem, to the derivation of a cost function, to the development and use of mathematical optimization techniques, to the design of features. In the present chapter, we review a number of fundamental ideas regarding mathematical functions—ideas that we will see used repeatedly throughout our study of machine learning. We also introduce common function notation and detail the form in which functions are most commonly seen in machine learning: as a table of values or a collection of data.

Different Representations of Mathematical Functions

To get an intuitive sense for what a mathematical function is, it is best to introduce the concept through a series of simple examples.

Example 3.1 (Historical Revenue of McDonald's) The table in the left panel of Fig. 3.1 shows a listing of the annual total revenue of the fast-food restaurant chain McDonald's over a period of 12 years from 2005 through 2016. This data consists of two columns: the *year* column and the *revenue* column. When presented with a table like this, we naturally scan across each

(continued)

R. Borhani et al., *Fundamentals of Machine Learning and Deep Learning in Medicine*, https://doi.org/10.1007/978-3-031-19502-0_3

Year	Revenue [$ billion]
2005	19.12
2006	20.90
2007	22.79
2008	23.52
2009	22.75
2010	24.08
2011	27.01
2012	27.57
2013	28.11
2014	27.44
2015	25.41
2016	26.42

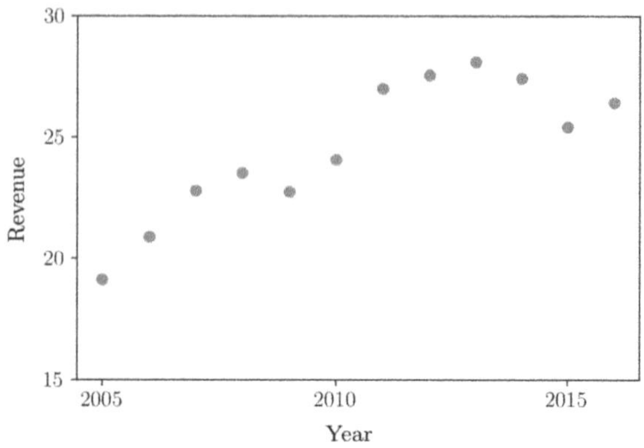

Fig. 3.1 Figure associated with Example 3.1. The annual total revenue of the fast-food restaurant chain McDonald's from 2005 to 2016. See text for further details

Example 3.1 (continued)
row to process its information. For example, in the year 2005, the revenue was 19.12 billion dollars, in 2006 the revenue was 22.90 billion dollars, and so on.

In processing this information, we start to understand the relationship between the *input value* (i.e., year) and the *output value* (i.e., revenue). We start to see each row as a *data point*, consisting of one input value and one output value, or taken together an input–output pair. For instance, the first row contains the data point or input–output pair (year, revenue) $=$ (2005, 19.12), the second row (year, revenue) $=$ (2006, 20.90), and so on.

While this might not be what you expect a "mathematical function" to look like, it is indeed one of the most common forms of functions we deal with in machine learning: a rule defining how input values and output values of a dataset or system relate to one another. In this example, the rule is explicit in the data itself: when the input (year) is 2005, the output (revenue) is 19.12 billion dollars, when the input is 2006, the output is 20.90 billion dollars, and so forth. In other words, here the phrase "mathematical function" simply means "a dataset consisting of input-output pairs."

We often plot such a mathematical function to make its relationship more visually explicit, as we have done in the right panel of Fig. 3.1 where each input–output pair from the data is drawn as a unique red circle. Since the input (year) is naturally ordered from smallest to largest, the plot can easily be related to the raw table of values on the left: points from the table, starting at the top and moving down, are plotted in the figure from left to right.

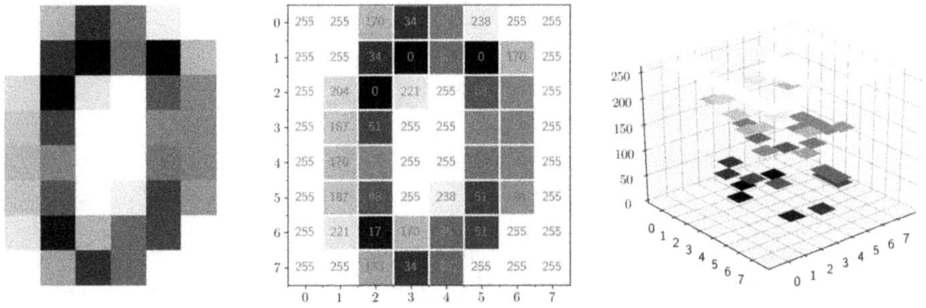

Fig. 3.2 Figure associated with Example 3.1. See text for details

Example 3.2 (The McDonald's Menu) A restaurant menu—like the one from McDonald's printed out in Table 3.1—provides a cornucopia of mathematical functions. Here, we have a dataset of food items, along with a large number of characteristics for each. Unlike the previous example, we no longer have a unique and easily identifiable input–output pair. For example, we could decide to look at the relationship between the food item and its allotment of calories, or the relationship between the food item and its total fat content. Notice, in either case (and unlike the previous example), the input is no longer numerical.

Example 3.3 (Digital Images) It is not always the case that a mathematical function comes in the form of a labeled table where input and output are placed neatly in separate columns. Take, for example, a standard grayscale image of the handwritten digit 0 shown in Fig. 3.2. The left panel displays the raw image itself, which is small enough that we can actually see all of the individual pixels that make it up.

Although we may not always think of them as one, a grayscale image is in fact a mathematical function. Recall from our discussion in Sect. "Imaging Data" that grayscale images are two-dimensional arrays of numbers (or matrices). This view of our digit image is plotted in the middle panel of Fig. 3.2 where we can see each pixel value printed in red on top of its respective pixel.

As a mathematical function, the grayscale image relates a pair of indices indicating a specific row and column of the array (the inputs) to a given pixel intensity value (the output). Therefore, we can write out this function as a table, as we have done in Table 3.2. Regardless of how we record them, each input–output pair in a grayscale image is a three-dimensional point. As such, we can plot any grayscale image as a surface in three-dimensional space. We do this for the digit image in the right panel of Fig. 3.2 where can visually examine how each input relates to its output.

Table 3.1 A subset of food items on the McDonald's menu along with each item's dietary information

Item	Calories	Fat	Sodium	Carbohydrates	Fiber	Sugars	Protein
McChicken	360	16	800	40	2	5	14
McRib	500	26	980	44	3	11	22
Big Mac	530	27	960	47	3	9	24
Filet-O-Fish	390	19	590	39	2	5	15
Cinnamon Melts	460	19	370	66	3	32	6
McDouble	380	17	840	34	2	7	22
Hamburger	240	8	480	32	1	6	12
Chicken McNuggets [4]	190	12	360	12	1	0	9
Chicken McNuggets [6]	280	18	540	18	1	0	13
Chicken McNuggets [40]	1880	118	3600	118	6	1	87
Hash Brown	150	9	310	15	2	0	1
Side Salad	20	0	10	4	1	2	1
Bacon Clubhouse Burger	720	40	1470	51	4	14	39
Buffalo Ranch McChicken	360	16	990	40	2	5	14
Daily Double	430	22	760	34	2	7	22
Cheeseburger	290	11	680	33	2	7	15
Fruit & Maple Oatmeal	290	4	160	58	5	32	5
Oatmeal Raisin Cookie	150	6	135	22	1	13	2
Egg McMuffin	300	13	750	31	4	3	17
Apple Slices	15	0	0	4	0	3	0
Small Mocha	340	11	150	49	2	42	10
Large Mocha	500	17	240	72	2	63	16
Bacon McDouble	440	22	1110	35	2	7	27
Jalapeño Double	430	23	1030	35	2	6	22
Baked Apple Pie	250	13	170	32	4	13	2
Crispy Ranch Snack Wrap	360	20	810	32	1	3	15
Grilled Ranch Snack Wrap	280	13	720	25	1	2	16
Sausage Burrito	300	16	790	26	1	2	12
Sausage McMuffin	370	23	780	29	4	2	14
Hot Fudge Sundae	330	9	170	53	1	48	8
Strawberry Sundae	280	6	85	49	0	45	6
Large French Fries	510	24	290	67	5	0	6
Hotcakes	350	9	590	60	3	14	8
Hot Caramel Sundae	340	8	150	60	0	43	7
Sausage McGriddles	420	22	1030	44	2	15	11
Small French Fries	230	11	130	30	2	0	2
Small Latte	170	9	115	15	1	12	9
Large Latte	280	14	180	24	1	20	15
Double Cheeseburger	430	21	1040	35	2	7	24
Steak & Egg McMuffin	430	23	960	31	4	3	26
Hotcakes & Sausage	520	24	930	61	3	14	15
Egg White Delight	250	8	770	30	4	3	18
Chocolate Chip Cookie	160	8	90	21	1	15	2
Quarter Pounder Deluxe	540	27	960	45	3	9	29
Sausage McMuffin + Egg	450	28	860	30	4	2	21
Sausage Biscuit	480	31	1190	39	3	3	11
Big Breakfast	740	48	1560	51	3	3	28

Table 3.2 The grayscale image in Fig. 3.2 represented as a table of input–output pairs

Input	Output	Input	Output	Input	Output	Input	Output
(0, 0)	255	(2, 0)	255	(4, 0)	255	(6, 0)	255
(0, 1)	255	(2, 1)	204	(4, 1)	170	(6, 1)	221
(0, 2)	170	(2, 2)	0	(4, 2)	119	(6, 2)	17
(0, 3)	34	(2, 3)	221	(4, 3)	255	(6, 3)	170
(0, 4)	102	(2, 4)	255	(4, 4)	255	(6, 4)	85
(0, 5)	238	(2, 5)	68	(4, 5)	102	(6, 5)	51
(0, 6)	255	(2, 6)	119	(4, 6)	119	(6, 6)	255
(0, 7)	255	(2, 7)	255	(4, 7)	255	(6, 7)	255
(1, 0)	255	(3, 0)	255	(5, 0)	255	(7, 0)	255
(1, 1)	255	(3, 1)	187	(5, 1)	187	(7, 1)	255
(1, 2)	34	(3, 2)	51	(5, 2)	68	(7, 2)	153
(1, 3)	0	(3, 3)	255	(5, 3)	255	(7, 3)	34
(1, 4)	85	(3, 4)	255	(5, 4)	238	(7, 4)	85
(1, 5)	0	(3, 5)	119	(5, 5)	51	(7, 5)	255
(1, 6)	170	(3, 6)	119	(5, 6)	136	(7, 6)	255
(1, 7)	255	(3, 7)	255	(5, 7)	255	(7, 7)	255

From what we have seen so far in the chapter, we can summarize a mathematical function as a *rule that relates inputs to outputs*. In a dataset, like the ones we encounter in the previous examples, this rule is *explicit*: it literally *is* the data itself. Sometimes (as with Example 3.2) we have to pluck out a mathematical function from a sea of choices, and sometimes (as with Example 3.3) the input–output relationship may not be clear at first sight. Nonetheless, mathematical functions abound. This omnipresence motivates the use of mathematical notation that allows us to more freely discuss functions at a higher level, categorize them by certain shared attributes, and build multi-use tools based on very general principles.

To denote the mathematical function relating an input x to an output y, we use the notation $y(x)$. For instance, in Example 3.2, we saw that the total revenue of the McDonald's corporation in year 2005 was 19.12 billion dollars, and we can therefore write $y(2010) = 19.12$. Similarly, in Example 3.3, we saw that the pixel intensity value at the top-left corner of the image was 255, and thus we can write $y(0, 0) = 255$.

In the remainder of this section, we review the classical way in which mathematical functions are typically described: using an algebraic equation or formula. In the process, we discuss how these functions implicitly produce datasets like the ones we have seen previously.

Take the familiar equation of a line

$$y(x) = -1 + \frac{1}{2}x \tag{3.1}$$

Input x	Output y
0	−1
3.6	0.8
2	0
−1	−1.5
2.5	0.25
6	2
−0.5	−1.25
−4	−3
5	1.5
−3.5	−2.75
⋮	⋮

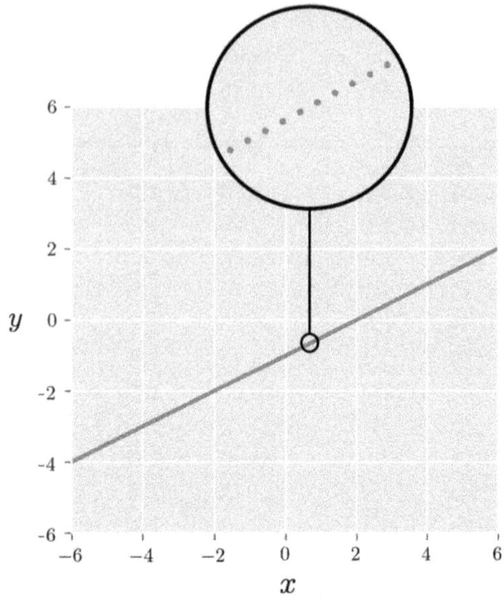

Fig. 3.3 (Left panel) Tabular view of the mathematical function $y(x) = -1 + \frac{1}{2}x$. It is impossible to list out every possible input–output pair in a table like this as there are infinitely many of them. (Right panel) The same function plotted over a small input range from $x = -6$ to $x = 6$

for instance. This is an explicitly written rule for taking an input x and transforming it into an associated output y. Writing down the equation of the line or any other formula gives us its rule *explicitly*: its recipe for transforming inputs into outputs. Note that with the algebraic formula for a mathematical function on hand, we can easily create its tabular view, as shown in the left panel of Fig. 3.3 for the function defined in (3.1). Here, the vertical dots in each column of the table indicate that we could keep on listing off input and output pairs (in no particular order). If we list out every possible input–output pair, this table would be equivalent to the equation defining it in (3.1)—albeit the list would be infinitely long!

Sometimes it is possible to visualize a mathematical function (when the input is only one- or two-dimensional). For example, in the right panel of Fig. 3.3, we show the plot of the mathematical function defined in (3.1). Although this plot appears to be continuous, it is not so in reality. If you could look closely enough, you would be able to see finely sampled but disjointed input–output pairs that make up the line. If we use a high enough sampling resolution, the plot will look continuous to the human eye, the way we might draw it using pencil and paper.

Which of the two modes of expressing a mathematical function better describes it: its algebraic equation or its equivalent tabular view consisting of all of its input–output pairs written out explicitly? To answer this question, note that if we have access to the former, we can always generate the latter—at least in theory by listing out every input–output pair using the equation to generate the pairs. But the reverse is not always true. If we only have access to a dataset/table describing a

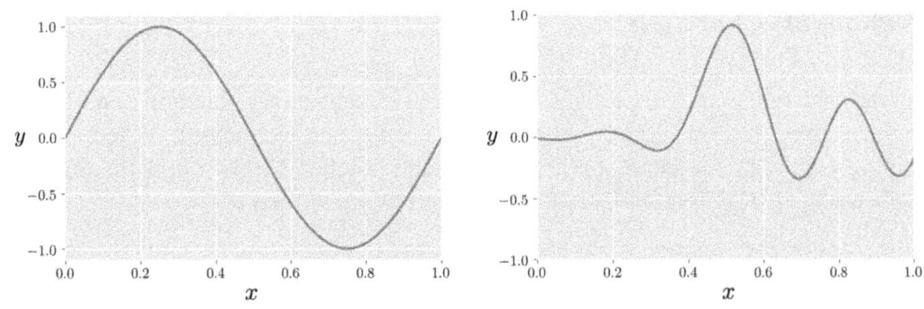

Fig. 3.4 Plots of two mathematical functions. Can you guess the algebraic equation generating each?

mathematical function (and not its algebraic expression), it is often not obvious how to draw conclusions vis-a-vis the associated algebraic form of the original function. We could attempt to plot the table of values, or some portion of it, as we did in Fig. 3.3, and intuit the equation $y = -1 + \frac{1}{2}x$ simply by looking at its plot. To see if this strategy works in general, we have plotted two more examples in Fig. 3.4. Take a moment to see if you can determine the algebraic equation of these plots using your visual intuition.

If you are familiar with elementary functions you may have been able to spot the equation for the example on the left, as

$$y(x) = \sin(2\pi x). \tag{3.2}$$

How about the second example on the right? Not many people—even if they are mathematicians—can correctly identify the function's underlying equation as

$$y(x) = e^{3x} \frac{\sin\left(24(x - 0.5)\right)}{120\,(x - 0.5)}. \tag{3.3}$$

The point here is that even when the input is only one-dimensional, identifying a function's equation by plotting some portion of its table of values is very difficult to do "by eye" alone. And, it is worth emphasizing that we could only even attempt this for functions of one or two inputs, since we cannot meaningfully visualize functions that take in three or more inputs.

Elementary Functions

In this section, we review elementary functions that are used extensively throughout not only the study of machine learning but many areas of science in general.

Polynomial Functions

Polynomial functions are perhaps the first set of elementary functions one learns about as they arise in virtually all areas of science and technology. When we are dealing with only one input, x, each polynomial function simply raises the input to a given power. The first few polynomial functions are written as

$$f_1(x) = x^1, \quad f_2(x) = x^2, \quad f_3(x) = x^3, \quad f_4(x) = x^4. \tag{3.4}$$

The first element in (3.4)—often written just as $f_1(x) = x$, ignoring the superscript 1)—is a simple line with a slope of 1 and a vertical intercept of 0, and the second, $f_2(x) = x^2$, a simple parabola. We can continue listing more polynomials, one for each positive integer k, with the kth polynomial taking the form $f_k(x) = x^k$. Because of this special indexing of powers, the polynomials naturally form a catalog or a family of functions. Of special interest to us in this book is the first member of this family that is the building block of linear machine learning models we study in great detail in Chaps. 4 and 5.

It is customary to define a degree-d polynomial as a linear combination of the first d polynomial functions (plus a constant term). For instance, $f(x) = 1+2x-3x^2+x^3$ is a degree-3 polynomial. In general, when we have N inputs $x_1, x_2, \ldots, x_N$, a polynomial function involves raising each input x_i to a nonzero integer power k_i and multiplying the result to form

$$f(x_1, x_2, \ldots, x_N) = x_1^{k_1} x_2^{k_2} \ldots x_N^{k_N}. \tag{3.5}$$

Several polynomial functions with one and two input(s) are plotted in the top and bottom panels of Fig. 3.5, respectively.

Reciprocal Functions

Reciprocal functions are created similarly to polynomial functions with one difference: instead of raising an input to a positive integer, we raise them to a negative one. The first few reciprocal functions are therefore written as

$$f_1(x) = x^{-1} = \frac{1}{x}, \quad f_2(x) = x^{-2} = \frac{1}{x^2}, \quad f_3(x) = x^{-3} = \frac{1}{x^3}, \tag{3.6}$$

and so on. Several examples of reciprocal functions are plotted in Fig. 3.6.

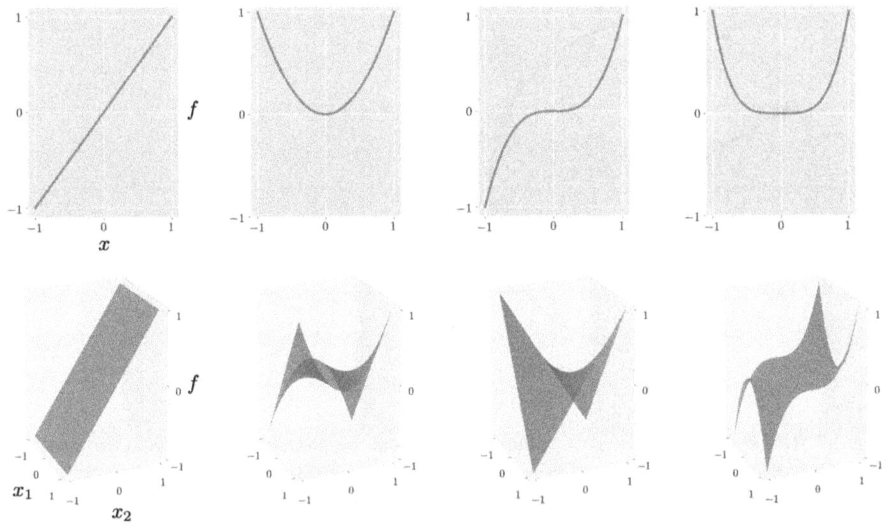

Fig. 3.5 Several polynomial functions. (Top panel) From left to right, the plot of $f(x) = x$, $f(x) = x^2$, $f(x) = x^3$, and $f(x) = x^4$. (Bottom panel) From left to right, the plot of $f(x_1, x_2) = x_2$, $f(x_1, x_2) = x_1 x_2^2$, $f(x_1, x_2) = x_1 x_2$, and $f(x_1, x_2) = x_1^2 x_2^3$

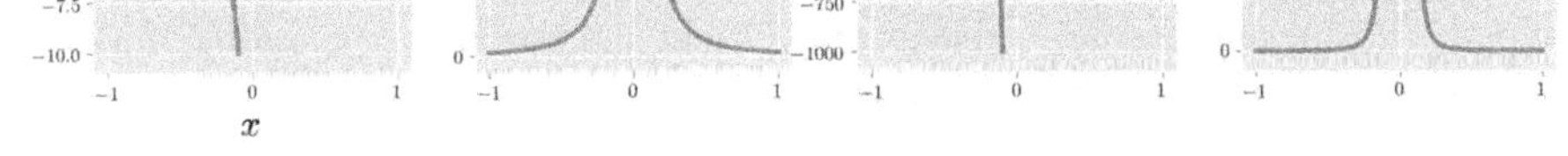

Fig. 3.6 Several reciprocal functions. From left to right, the plot of $f(x) = x^{-1}$, $f(x) = x^{-2}$, $f(x) = x^{-3}$, and $f(x) = x^{-4}$

Trigonometric and Hyperbolic Functions

The basic trigonometric functions are derived from the simple relations of a right triangle and take on a repeating wave-like shape. The first of these are the sine and cosine functions written, respectively, for a scalar input x as $\sin(x)$ and $\cos(x)$. These two elementary functions originate in tracking the vertical and horizontal coordinates of a single point on the unit circle

$$x^2 + y^2 = 1 \tag{3.7}$$

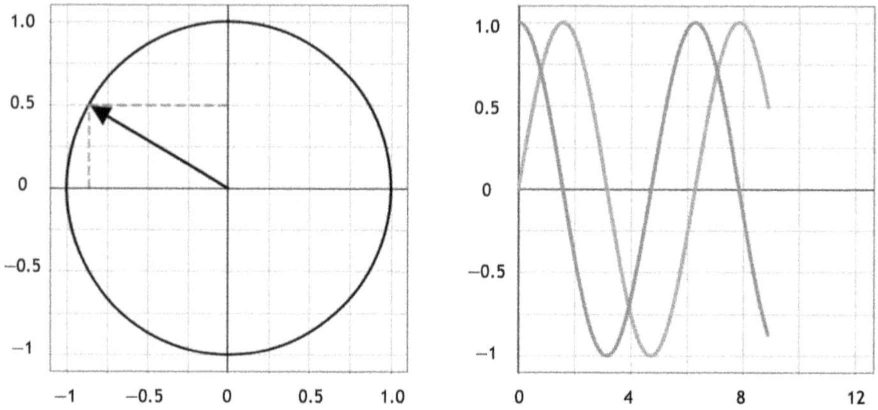

Fig. 3.7 The sine (red) and cosine (blue) functions can be plotted by tracking the vertical and horizontal position of the endpoint of an arrow stemming from the origin and ending on the unit circle as the endpoint moves counterclockwise. Every time the endpoint completes one loop around the circle each function naturally repeats itself, making sine and cosine *periodic* functions

as it smoothly moves counterclockwise around, as illustrated in Fig. 3.7.

Historically, the sine and cosine functions have been used to model the (periodic) movements of celestial bodies. Other common trigonometric functions are based on various ratios of these two fundamental functions. For example, the tangent function is defined as the ratio of sine to cosine, that is, $\tan(x) = \frac{\sin(x)}{\cos(x)}$. Sine and cosine functions for two inputs (x_1 and x_2) involve creating wave elements in each variable individually and multiplying the result, with a similar pattern holding for general N-dimensional input as well.

In analogy to trigonometric functions, the basic hyperbolic functions—called hyperbolic sine and cosine—arise as the vertical and horizontal positions of a point tracing out the unit hyperbola given by

$$x^2 - y^2 = 1. \tag{3.8}$$

Other common hyperbolic functions are based on various ratios of these two fundamental functions. For example, the hyperbolic tangent function is defined as the ratio of hyperbolic sine to hyperbolic cosine, that is, $\tanh(x) = \frac{\sinh(x)}{\cosh(x)}$.

Exponential Functions

A well-known Indian folktale tells the story of a king who enjoyed inviting people to play Chess against him. One day the king offered to grant a traveling savant whatever reward he wanted if he beat the king in the game. The savant agreed, but demanded the king pay him in a rather strange way: if the savant won, the king

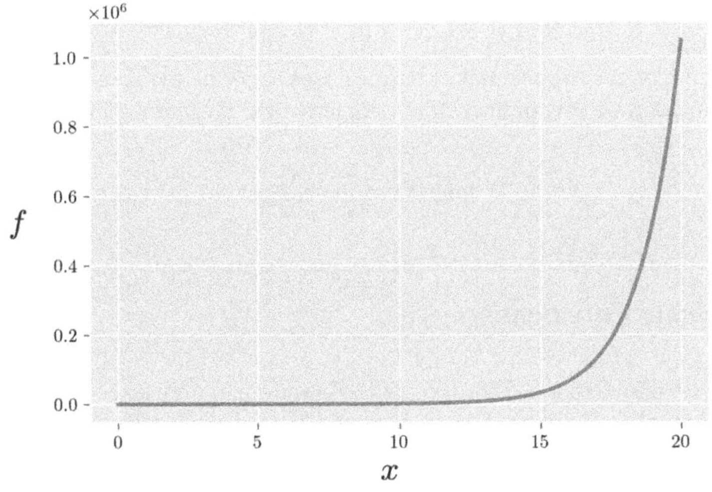

Fig. 3.8 Plot of the exponential function $f(x) = 2^x$

would put a single grain of rice on the first square of the Chessboard and double it on every consequent one. The two played and the savant won.

The king ordered a large bag of rice to be brought in and started placing the grains according to the mutually agreed upon arrangement: one grain on the first square, two on the second, four on the third, and so on and so forth. By the time he reached the 21st square, he had already emptied the entire bag. Soon the king realized all the rice in his entire kingdom would not be enough to fulfill his pledge to the savant.

The king in this fable failed to appreciate the incredibly rapid growth of the exponential function $f(x) = 2^x$, plotted in Fig. 3.8. In general, an exponential function can be defined for any base value. For example, $f(x) = 10^x$ defines an exponential with base 10.

Another widely used choice for the base value is the Euler's number denoted $e = 2.71828\ldots$, where the decimal expansion is unending and non-repeating. This number—credited to seventeenth century mathematician Jacob Bernoulli—originally arose out of a thought experiment posed about compound interest payments. Suppose we have a principal of \$1.00 in the bank and receive 100% interest from the bank per year, credited once at the end of the year. This means we would double our amount of money after one year, i.e., we multiply our principal by 2. Notice what changes if instead of receiving one interest payment of 100% on our principal we received 2 payments of 50% interest during the year. At the first crediting, we multiply the principal by 1.5 (to get 50% interest). However, at the second crediting, we multiply this *updated* value by 1.5, or in other words, we multiply our principal by $(1.5)^2 = (1+\frac{1}{2})^2$. If we keep going in this way, supposing we credit $33.33\ldots\%$ interest 3 times per year, we end up multiplying the principal by $(1 + \frac{1}{3})^3$, cutting the interest in quarters we end up multiplying the principal by $(1 + \frac{1}{4})^4$, etc. In general, if we cut the interest payments into n equal pieces, we multiply the principal by $(1+\frac{1}{n})^n$. It is this quantity—as n grows to infinity—that converges to e.

Interestingly, the exponential of base e arises as a way to express the hyperbolic tangent function we saw in Sect. “Trigonometric and Hyperbolic Functions”, as

$$\tanh(x) = \frac{e^x - e^{-x}}{e^x + e^{-x}}. \tag{3.9}$$

Logarithmic Functions

What is $810,456,018 \times 6,388,100,279$? Nowadays, it only takes a few seconds to type these numbers into a trusty calculator and find the answer. But before the advent of calculators, one had no choice but to multiplying two large numbers like these by hand: an obviously tedious and time-consuming task, requiring careful book keeping to avoid clerical errors. Necessity being the mother of all invention however, people invented all sorts of tricks to make this sort of computations easier.

The logarithm—first invented to cut big multiplication problems down to size by turning multiplication into addition—is an elementary function with a wide range of modern applications. Based on the exponential function with generic base b, the logarithm of base b is defined as

$$y = \log_b(x) \iff b^y = x. \tag{3.10}$$

Using this definition, one can quickly verify that indeed this function (regardless of the choice of base b) turns multiplication into addition. The logarithm and exponential functions are inverses of one another. This allowed one to take the multiplication of two large numbers p and q, and instead of doing this multiplication, evaluating p and q by the logarithm (usually looking up the values $\log_b(p)$ and $\log_b(q)$ values in a table), adding the result, and then exponentiating to get the resulting product $p \cdot q$. The logarithm function with base e (the Euler’s number) is commonly referred to as the natural logarithm and is plotted in Fig. 3.9. When dealing with natural logarithm, it is commonplace (for the sake of brevity) to drop the base e from the notation and write the natural logarithm function simply as $f(x) = \log(x)$.

Step Functions

Compared with the previous functions that were defined by a single equation over their entire input domain, step functions are defined in cases over subregions of their input. Over each subregion, the step functions are constant but can take on different values on each subregion. For example, a step function with two steps has the algebraic form

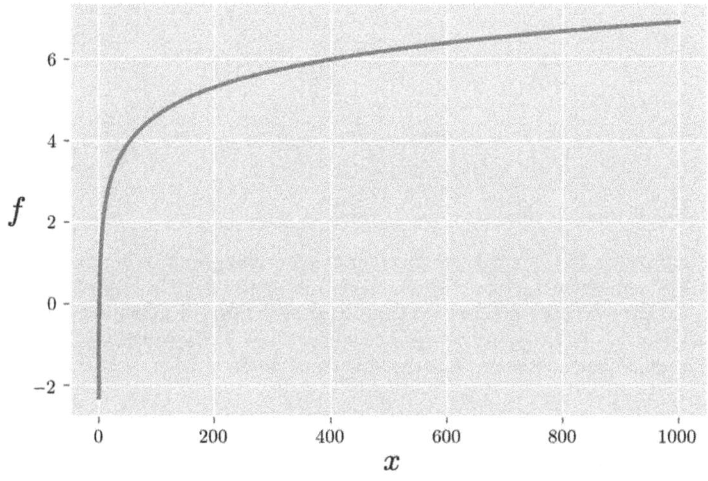

Fig. 3.9 Plot of the logarithmic function $f(x) = \log(x)$

$$f(x) = \begin{cases} v_1 & \text{if } x < s \\ v_2 & \text{if } x > s \end{cases}, \tag{3.11}$$

where s is referred to as a *split point*, and v_1 and v_2 are two constant values. Typically, the value of the function at the split point $x = s$ is not of great significance and is often set as the average of v_1 and v_2, i.e., $f(s) = \frac{v_1+v_2}{2}$. The sign function is a prime and often used example of a step function where $s = 0$, $v_1 = -1$, and $v_2 = +1$. In general, a step function with N steps breaks the input into N subregions, taking on a different value over each subregion

$$f(x) = \begin{cases} v_1 & \text{if } x < s_1 \\ v_2 & \text{if } s_1 < x < s_2 \\ \vdots & \vdots \\ v_{N-1} & \text{if } s_{N-2} < x < s_{N-1} \\ v_N & \text{if } s_{N-1} < x \end{cases} \tag{3.12}$$

and hence has $N - 1$ split points s_1 through s_{N-1}, with N constant levels denoted v_1 through v_N.

Many analog (continuous) signals such as radio and television signals often look like some sort of sine function when broadcast. At the receiver, however, an electronic device will digitize (or quantize) such signals, which entails transforming the original wavy analog signal into a step function that closely resembles it. By doing so, far fewer values are required to store and process the signal (just the

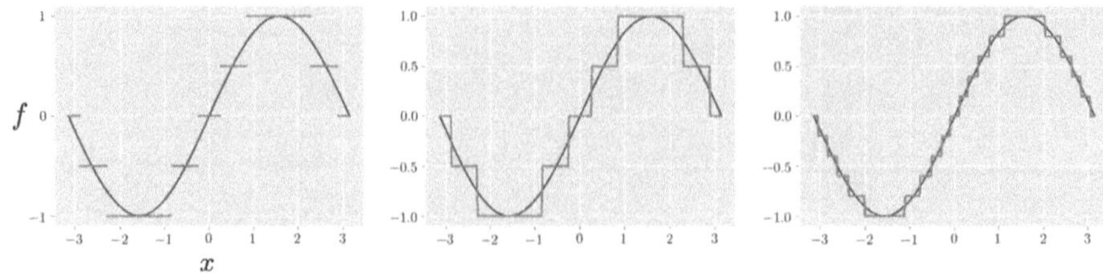

Fig. 3.10 (Left panel) The original sine function in black along with its digitized version (a step function with 9 levels/steps) in red. (Middle panel) A more common way of plotting the step function on the left where all the discontinuities have been filled in so that the step function can be visualized more easily. (Right panel) As the number of levels/steps increases, the step function resembles the underlying continuous sine function more closely

values of the steps and splitting points, as opposed to the entire original function). Figure 3.10 illustrates a facsimile of this idea for a simple sine function.

Elementary Operations

In this section, we discuss a number of ways to adjust the elementary functions introduced in Sect. "Elementary Functions" as well as various ways of combining these elementary functions to create an unending array of interesting and complicated mathematical functions with known algebraic equations.

Basic Function Adjustments

Multiplying a function $f(x)$ by a scalar weight w results in a new function $w \cdot f(x)$ that is an amplified version of the original $f(x)$ when $w > 1$. This is essentially what an electronic amplifier does to its input signal. When $0 < w < 1$, on the other hand, the resulting function would be an attenuated version of $f(x)$. In the special case where $w = -1$, the result is simply the reflection of $f(x)$ over the horizontal axis.

Multiplying the input to $f(x)$ by a scalar weight w results in a new function $f(wx)$ that is a shrunk version (along the horizontal axis) of the original $f(x)$ when $w > 1$. When $0 < w < 1$, on the other hand, the resulting function would be a stretched version of $f(x)$. In the special case where $w = -1$, the result is simply the reflection of $f(x)$ over the vertical axis.

Finally, adding a scalar weight w to the function $f(x)$ simply elevates its plot by w units along the vertical axis. Adding w to the input x, on the other hand, causes $f(x)$ to move along the horizontal axis. These basic adjustments are illustrated in Fig. 3.11.

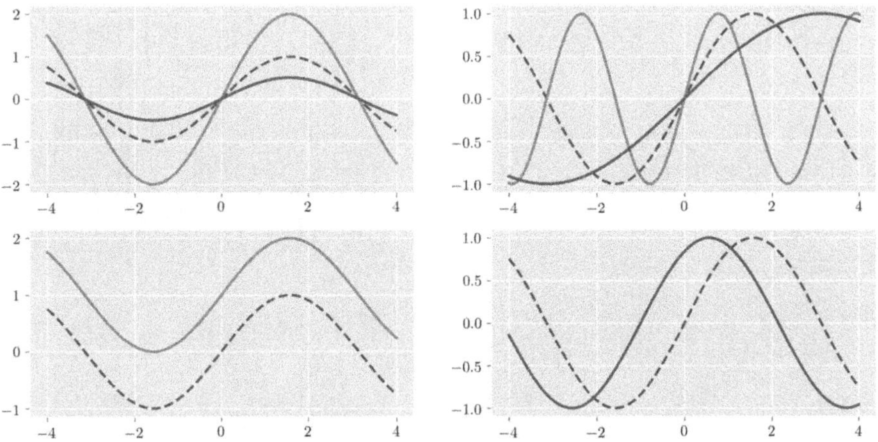

Fig. 3.11 Illustration of various function adjustments including amplification, attenuation, squeezing, stretching, as well as horizontal and vertical shifts. The original function $f(x) = \sin(x)$ is drawn in dashed black for comparison. (Top-left panel) Plots of the functions $2f(x)$ and $\frac{1}{2}f(x)$ shown in red and blue, respectively, to exemplify function amplification and attenuation. (Top-right panel) Plots of the functions $f(2x)$ and $f(\frac{1}{2}x)$ shown in red and blue, respectively, to exemplify squeezing and stretching. (Bottom-left panel) Plot of the function $f(x) + 1$ (in red) exemplifies a vertical shift. (Bottom-right panel) Plot of the function $f(x + 1)$ (in blue) exemplifies a horizontal shift

Addition and Multiplication of Functions

Just like numbers, basic arithmetic operations including addition (or subtraction) and multiplication (or division) can be used to combine two (or more) functions as well. For instance, $f_1(x) + f_2(x)$ is a new function formed by adding the values of $f_1(x)$ and $f_2(x)$ at each point over their entire common domain.

Akin to addition, we can define multiplication of two functions $f_1(x)$ and $f_2(x)$ denoted by $f_1(x) \times f_2(x)$, or just simply $f_1(x)\,f_2(x)$. Interestingly, amplitude modulation (AM) radio broadcasting was invented in the early 1900 based on the simple idea of multiplying a message signal by a sinusoidal function (called the carrier signal) at the transmitter side. Amplitude modulation makes it possible to broadcast multiple messages simultaneously over a shared medium (or channel). Function addition and multiplication are illustrated in Fig. 3.12.

Composition of Functions

Another common way of combining two functions is by *composing* them. Simply speaking, this means that we take the output of one function and use it as input to the other. Take functions x^3 and $\sin(x)$, for example. We can plug x^3 into $\sin(x)$ to

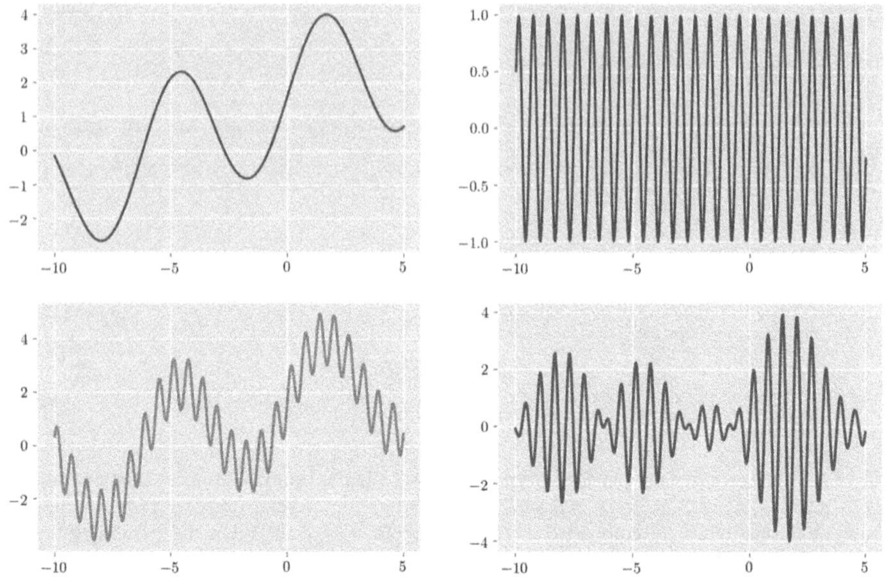

Fig. 3.12 Illustration of function addition and multiplication using the functions $f_1(x) = 2\sin(x) + 3\cos(\frac{1}{10}x - 1)$ and $f_2(x) = \sin(10x)$ plotted in the top-left panel and the top-right panel, respectively. The addition of the two functions, $f_1(x) + f_2(x)$, is plotted in the bottom-left panel, and the multiplication of the two functions, $f_1(x) \times f_2(x)$, is plotted in the bottom-right panel

get $\sin\left(x^3\right)$, or alternatively, we can plug the sine function into the cubic one to get $(\sin(x))^3$.

Importantly, the order in which we compose the two functions is important. This is different from what we saw with addition or multiplication, where we always have $x^3 + \sin(x) = \sin(x) + x^3$, and similarly, $x^3 \times \sin(x) = \sin(x) \times x^3$. This gives composition, as a way of combining functions, much more flexibility compared to addition or multiplication, especially when dealing with more than two functions. Let us verify this observation by adding a third function to the mix: the exponential e^x. While again there is only one way to combine x^3, $\sin(x)$, and e^x via addition (i.e., $x^3 + \sin(x) + e^x$) or multiplication (i.e., $x^3 \times \sin(x) \times e^x$), we have now many different ways to compose these three functions: we can select any of the three, plug it into one of the two remaining functions, take the result, and plug it into the last one. Figure 3.13 shows the functions resulted from all $3! = 3 \times 2 \times 1$ ways in which we can compose these three functions.

Notationally, the composition of $f_1(x)$ with $f_2(x)$ is written as $f_1(f_2(x))$, and in general, we have that

$$f_1(f_2(x)) \neq f_2(f_1(x)). \tag{3.13}$$

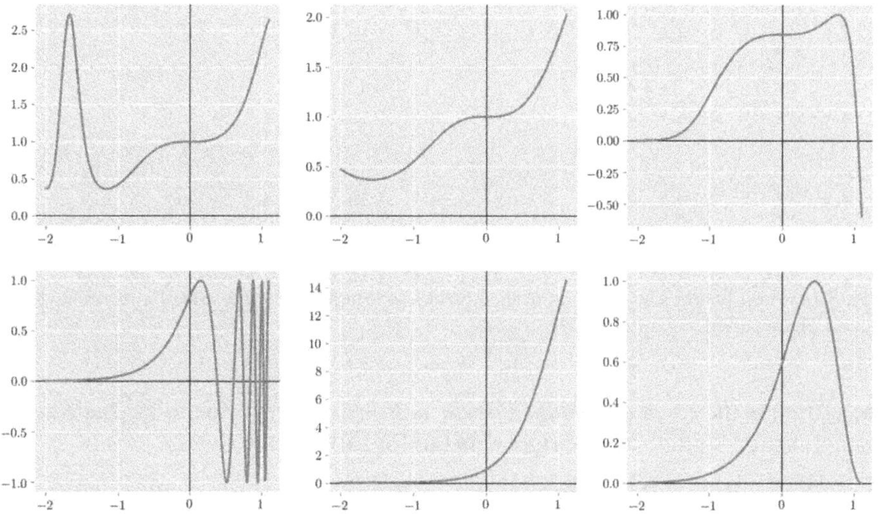

Fig. 3.13 Six different ways of composing three elementary functions: $f_1(x) = x^3$, $f_2(x) = \sin(x)$, and $f_3(x) = e^x$. (Top-left panel) Plot of the function $f_3(f_2(f_1(x))) = e^{\sin(x^3)}$. (Top-middle panel) Plot of the function $f_3(f_1(f_2(x))) = e^{\sin^3(x)}$. (Top-right panel) Plot of the function $f_2(f_3(f_1(x))) = \sin\left(e^{x^3}\right)$. (Bottom-left panel) Plot of the function $f_2(f_1(f_3(x))) = \sin\left((e^x)^3\right)$. (Bottom-middle panel) Plot of the function $f_1(f_3(f_2(x))) = \left(e^{\sin(x)}\right)^3$. (Bottom-right panel) Plot of the function $f_1(f_2(f_3(x))) = (\sin(e^x))^3$

Min–Max Operations

The maximum of two functions $f_1(x)$ and $f_2(x)$, denoted by $\max(f_1(x), f_2(x))$, is formed by setting the output to the larger value of $f_1(x)$ and $f_2(x)$ for every x in the common domain of $f_1(x)$ and $f_2(x)$. The minimum of two functions is defined in a similar manner, only this time by setting the output to the smaller value of the two. The following is a practical use case of this function operation from the field of electrical engineering.

Electricity is delivered to the point of consumption in AC (Alternating Current) mode, meaning that the voltage you get at your outlet is a sinusoidal waveform with both positive and negative cycles. This is while virtually every electronic device (mobile phone, laptop, etc.) operates on DC (direct current) power and thus requires a constant steady supply of voltage. A conversion from AC to DC therefore has to take place inside the power adapter: this is the function of a rectifier. In its simplest form, the rectifier comprises a single diode that blocks negative cycles of the AC waveform and only allows positive cycles to pass. The diode's output voltage f_{out} can then be expressed in terms of the input voltage f_{in} as $f_{\text{out}}(x) = \max(0, f_{\text{in}}(x))$.

In the left panel of Fig. 3.14, we show the shape of $f_{\text{out}}(x)$ when the input is a simple sine function $f_{\text{in}}(x) = \sin(x)$. When $f_{\text{in}}(x) = x$, the output $f_{\text{out}}(x) =$

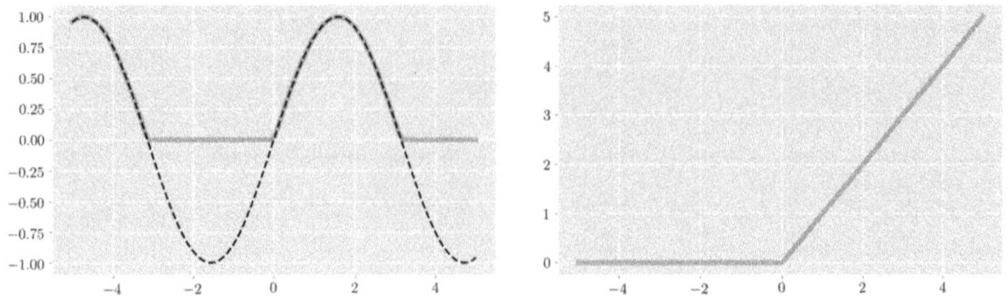

Fig. 3.14 (Left panel) The input (in dashed black) and output (in solid red) of a rectifier. (Right panel) The rectified linear unit

max $(0, x)$ is the so-called *rectified linear unit*—also known due to its shape as the ramp function—plotted in the right panel of Fig. 3.14.

Constructing Complex Functions Using Elementary Functions and Operations

In Sects. "Elementary Functions" and "Elementary Operations", we reviewed elementary mathematical functions (e.g., trigonometric functions, exponential functions, etc.) and operations (e.g., addition, multiplication, composition, etc.). These elementary functions and operations—summarized in Tables 3.3 and 3.4, respectively—can be combined in order to construct new functions of arbitrary complexity. Take the function

$$f(x) = \frac{\cos(16x)}{1 + x^2} \tag{3.14}$$

for instance, whose plot is shown in the left panel of Fig. 3.15. It is easy to verify that this seemingly complex function was created using only the elementary functions and operations in Tables 3.3 and 3.4, according to the graphical recipe shown in the right panel of Fig. 3.15.

Problems

3.1 A Valid Function or Not?

As we saw throughout the chapter, a mathematical function is any rule connecting an input to an output. While two (or more) distinct input values can share the same common output value, the converse is not true: one input cannot generate more than

Table 3.3 A (non-exhaustive) list of elementary mathematical functions

Row	Elementary function	Algebraic notation
1	The constant function	$f(x) = c$
2	The identity function	$f(x) = x$
3	The sine function	$f(x) = \sin(x)$
4	The cosine function	$f(x) = \cos(x)$
5	The exponential function	$f(x) = e^x$
6	The natural log function	$f(x) = \log(x)$
7	The rectified linear unit (ReLU) function	$f(x) = \max(0, x)$
⋮	⋮	⋮

Table 3.4 A (non-exhaustive) list of elementary function operations

Row	Elementary operation	Algebraic notation
1	Addition of $f_1(x)$ and $f_2(x)$	$f_1(x) + f_2(x)$
2	Multiplication of $f_1(x)$ and $f_2(x)$	$f_1(x) \cdot f_2(x)$
3	Division of $f_1(x)$ by $f_2(x)$	$\frac{f_1(x)}{f_2(x)}$
4	Composition of $f_1(x)$ with $f_2(x)$	$f_1(f_2(x))$
⋮	⋮	⋮

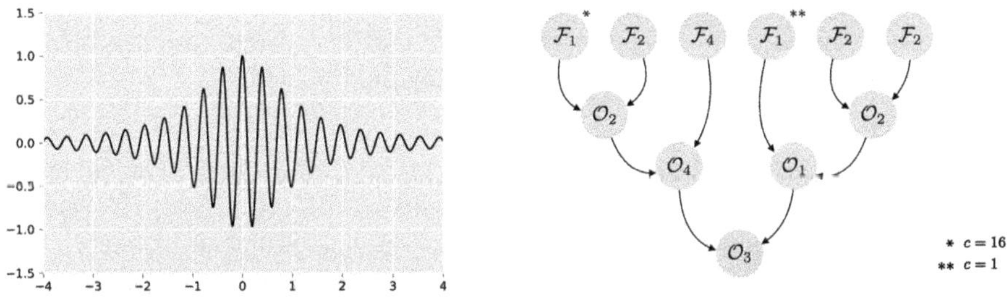

Fig. 3.15 (Left panel) The plot of the function $f(x) = \frac{\cos(16x)}{1+x^2}$. (Right panel) A graphical representation of how the elementary functions and operations in Tables 3.3 and 3.4 can be combined to form $f(x)$. Here, $\mathcal{F}_i$ denotes the elementary function in the ith row of Table 3.3, and O_j denotes the elementary operation in the jth row of Table 3.4

one output. With this definition in mind, determine whether each of the following input–output relationships defines a valid function:

(a) The relationship between a food item (input) and its sodium content (output), as provided in Table 3.1
(b) The relationship between the amount of protein in a food item (input) and its total calories (output), as provided in Table 3.1
(c) The relationship between x (input) and y (output), defined through the equation $2x + 3y + xy = 1$
(d) The relationship between x (input) and y (output), defined through the equation $x^2 + y^2 = xy$

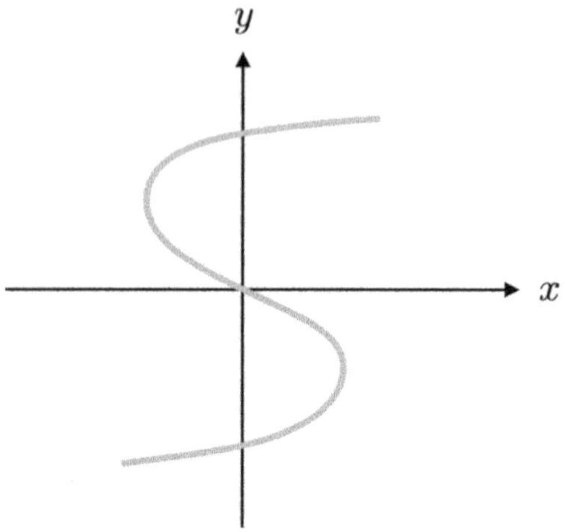

Fig. 3.16 Figure associated with Exercise 3.1

(e) The relationship between x (input) and y (output), captured in the s-shaped plot shown in Fig. 3.16

3.2 Multiplication of Large Numbers
Use the definition in (3.10) to show how two very large numbers can be multiplied together via addition, without invoking multiplication.

3.3 Basic Function Adjustments
Figure 3.11 illustrates how various basic adjustments (e.g., amplification, attenuation, squeezing, stretching, etc.) change the shape of a given function. Starting with the cosine function $f(x) = \cos(x)$, use these basic adjustments to create a new trigonometric function whose output is always bounded between -0.2 and $+0.3$, and whose plot pierces the horizontal axis exactly 3 times over the unit interval, i.e., when $0 \leq x \leq 1$.

3.4 The Inverse Function
A function $g(x)$ is said to be the inverse of $f(x)$ if the composition of the two always equals 1, that is, $g(f(x)) = 1$. Determine the inverse function for each of the following functions:

(a) $f(x) = x$.
(b) $f(x) = e^x$.
(c) $f(x) = e^{10x}$.

3.5 Construction of Endlessly Complex Functions from Elementary Building Blocks
In Sect. "Constructing Complex Functions Using Elementary Functions and Operations", we showed how the function $f(x) = \frac{\cos(16x)}{1+x^2}$ can be constructed using the elementary functions and operations listed in Tables 3.3 and 3.4. In this exercise, you show this construction may be done for each of the functions provided below,

by producing a similar graphical representation to the one shown in the right panel of Fig. 3.15.

(a) $f(x) = 1 + x^2 + x^4$.
(b) $f(x) = \tanh(x) = \frac{e^x - e^{-x}}{e^x + e^{-x}}$.
(c) $f(x) = \log\left(\frac{1}{1+e^{-x}}\right)$.

Chapter 4
Linear Regression

A large number of our day-to-day experiences and activities are governed by linear phenomena. For instance, the distance traveled by a car at a certain speed is linearly related to the duration of the trip. When an object is thrown, its acceleration is a linear function of the amount of force exerted to throw the object. The sales tax owed on a purchased item changes linearly with the item's original price. The recommended dosages for many medications are linear functions of the patient's weight. And, the list goes on.

Linear regression is the machine learning task of uncovering the hidden linear relationship between the input and output data. In this chapter, we study linear regression from the ground up, laying the foundation for discussion of more complex nonlinear models in the chapters to come.

Linear Regression with One-Dimensional Input

We start our discussion of linear regression by studying a very simple regression dataset consisting only of four input–output pairs

$$\begin{aligned}(x_1, y_1) &= (0, -1),\\ (x_2, y_2) &= (2, 0),\\ (x_3, y_3) &= (4, 1),\\ (x_4, y_4) &= (6, 2),\end{aligned} \tag{4.1}$$

Supplementary Information The online version contains supplementary material available at (https://doi.org/10.1007/978-3-031-19502-0_4).

R. Borhani et al., *Fundamentals of Machine Learning and Deep Learning in Medicine*, https://doi.org/10.1007/978-3-031-19502-0_4

where the first element of each pair is a sample input and the second element is the corresponding output. Before proceeding any further, take a moment and try to solve this regression problem yourself by finding a mathematical relationship (whether linear or nonlinear) that could explain this data. In other words, use your mathematical intuition to find a function $f(\cdot)$ such that

$$\begin{aligned} f(0) &= -1, \\ f(2) &= 0, \\ f(4) &= 1, \\ f(6) &= 2. \end{aligned} \tag{4.2}$$

If you have not managed to find a solution already, you may find it helpful to plot this data (as we have done in Fig. 4.1) and inspect it visually. Do you see a trend or pattern emerge?

Most (if not all) people would immediately recognize a linear relationship between the input and output in this case, even though countless other (nonlinear) functions satisfying the equations in (4.2) also exist. The trigonometric function $f(x) = \sin^2(\frac{\pi}{4}x) - \sin(\frac{\pi}{4}x) - \cos(\frac{\pi}{4}x)$ is one example.

The reason why we are quicker to pick a linear solution over a nonlinear one can be explained by the *ubiquity* and *simplicity* of linear functions. As discussed earlier in the introduction to the chapter, we are surrounded by linear phenomena, and as a result, our brains have evolved to recognize linearity with ease. Moreover, the *Occam's razor* principle states that when presented with competing hypotheses with identical prediction power, the simplest solution is always preferable. In the words of the second century AD Greek mathematician Claudius Ptolemy "in general, we consider it a good principle to explain a phenomenon by the simplest hypothesis possible."

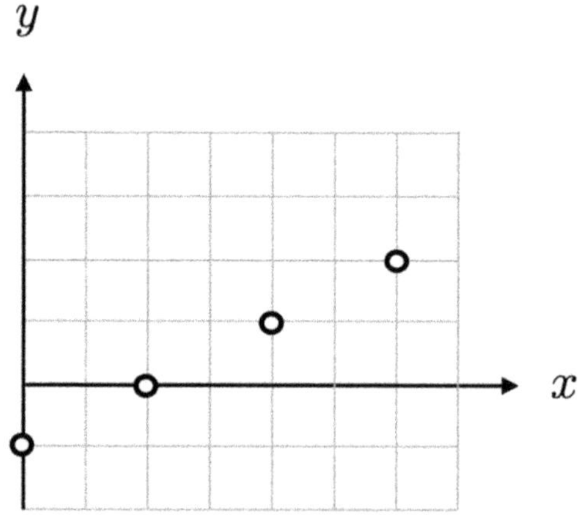

Fig. 4.1 The plot of the regression dataset in (4.1) where all four data points appear to be lying on a straight line. See text for further details

Linear functions are the simplest of all mathematical functions, both algebraically and geometrically, making them easy for humans to understand, intuit, interpret, and wield. A linear function with one-dimensional input takes the general form of

$$f(x) = w_0 + w_1 x, \tag{4.3}$$

where the parameter w_0 represents the function's *bias* (or vertical intercept) and the parameter w_1 represents its *slope* (or rise over run). Solving a linear regression problem then becomes synonymous with finding the correct values for w_0 and w_1 in a way that all equations in (4.2) hold.

Substituting the parametric expression of $f(\cdot)$ in (4.3) into (4.2), we have

$$\begin{aligned} w_0 \quad\quad &= -1, \\ w_0 + 2w_1 &= 0, \\ w_0 + 4w_1 &= 1, \\ w_0 + 6w_1 &= 2. \end{aligned} \tag{4.4}$$

This linear system of equations has a unique solution given by $(w_0, w_1) = (-1, \frac{1}{2})$, which yields $f(x) = -1 + \frac{1}{2}x$ as the linear model underlying the regression dataset in (4.1).

The Least Squares Cost Function

The regression datasets encountered in practice differ from the previously studied toy dataset in (4.1) in two important ways. First, real-world datasets are typically much larger in size, some having in excess of millions of data points. Therefore, from this point on, we assume regression datasets consist, in general, of p input–output pairs where p can be arbitrarily large. The general setup for linear regression problems can then be cast as a set of p linear equations, written compactly as

$$w_0 + w_1 x_i = y_i, \qquad i = 1, 2, \ldots, p. \tag{4.5}$$

Second, and perhaps more importantly, there is no guarantee for all p data points in a given regression dataset to be *collinear*, meaning that they all fall precisely on a single straight line. In fact, it is highly unlikely to encounter fully collinear datasets in real-life settings even if the underlying relationship between the input and output is truly linear. This is because a certain amount of noise is always present in the data as a result of various types of observational and measurement errors that cannot be eliminated entirely. Mathematically speaking, this means that the linear system of equations in (4.5) will almost never have any solutions if the presence of noise is not taken into account.

We can model the existence of noise by adding a new variable ϵ_i to the output y_i in (4.5) to form the following "noisy" system of equations:

$$w_0 + w_1 x_i = y_i + \epsilon_i, \qquad i = 1, 2, \ldots, p. \tag{4.6}$$

Note, however, that with this adjustment the linear system above has now more unknown variables ($p + 2$) than equations (p), causing it to have infinitely many solutions. Thus, a new strategy is needed to solve (4.6) to retrieve the optimal values for w_0 and w_1.

Rearranging (4.6) by bringing the term y_i to the left hand side and squaring both sides yield an equivalent system of equations

$$(w_0 + w_1 x_i - y_i)^2 = \epsilon_i^2, \qquad i = 1, 2, \ldots, p, \tag{4.7}$$

in which the noise/error terms are now isolated from the rest of the variables. In addition, by squaring both sides, we can make sure that both positive and negative error values of the same magnitude contribute equally to the *mean squared error* (or MSE) defined, over the whole dataset, as

$$\text{MSE} = \frac{1}{p} \sum_{i=1}^{p} \epsilon_i^2. \tag{4.8}$$

Ideally, we would want the MSE to be 0. However, this implies that all ϵ_i's should be zero, which, as stated previously, is not a practical possibility. If we cannot vanish the mean squared error entirely, the next best thing we could do is to make it as small as possible. This desire forms the basis of the *least squares* framework, depicted visually in Fig. 4.2, in which we determine the optimal values for w_0 and w_1 by minimizing the least squares cost function

$$g(w_0, w_1) = \frac{1}{p} \sum_{i=1}^{p} \epsilon_i^2 = \frac{1}{p} \sum_{i=1}^{p} (w_0 + w_1 x_i - y_i)^2. \tag{4.9}$$

Minimizing the least squares cost function in (4.9) is no herculean task and can be done by setting the partial derivative of $g(\cdot)$ to 0 with respect to its inputs. The partial derivative of $g(\cdot)$ with respect to w_0 can be written, and simplified, as

$$\frac{\partial g}{\partial w_0} = \frac{1}{p} \sum_{i=1}^{p} 2\,(w_0 + w_1 x_i - y_i) \frac{\partial (w_0 + w_1 x_i - y_i)}{\partial w_0} = \frac{2}{p} \sum_{i=1}^{p} (w_0 + w_1 x_i - y_i). \tag{4.10}$$

Similarly, the partial derivative of $g(\cdot)$ with respect to w_1 can be written, and simplified, as

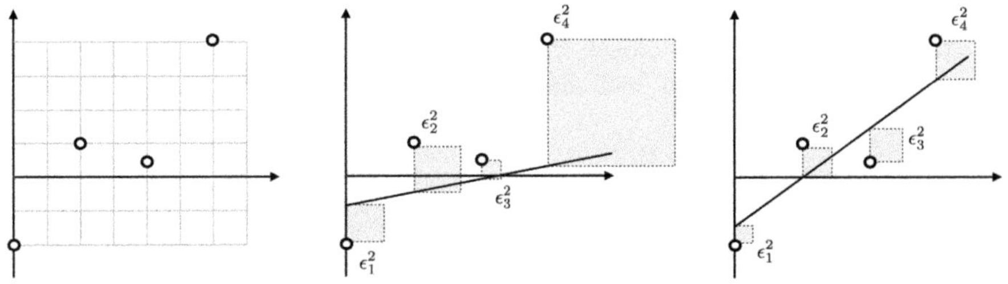

Fig. 4.2 (Left panel) A noisy version of the toy regression dataset shown originally in Fig. 4.1. Note that with the addition of noise the data points no longer lie on a straight line. (Middle panel) A "bad" linear model for fitting this data produces relatively large squared error values. Here, the ith square has an area equal to ϵ_i^2. (Right panel) A "good" linear model should produce relatively small squared error values overall. Visually speaking, the least squares framework seeks out the linear model producing the least average amount of the gray color

$$\frac{\partial g}{\partial w_1} = \frac{1}{p}\sum_{i=1}^{p} 2\left(w_0 + w_1 x_i - y_i\right)\frac{\partial\left(w_0 + w_1 x_i - y_i\right)}{\partial w_1} = \frac{2}{p}\sum_{i=1}^{p}(w_0 + w_1 x_i - y_i)x_i. \tag{4.11}$$

Setting (4.10) and (4.11) to zero and applying simple algebraic rearrangements lead to the following linear system of equations

$$\begin{aligned} w_0\, p + w_1 \sum_{i=1}^{p} x_i &= \sum_{i=1}^{p} y_i, \\ w_0 \sum_{i=1}^{p} x_i + w_1 \sum_{i=1}^{p} x_i^2 &= \sum_{i=1}^{p} y_i x_i, \end{aligned} \tag{4.12}$$

which can be written in matrix format as

$$\begin{bmatrix} p & \sum_{i=1}^{p} x_i \\ \sum_{i=1}^{p} x_i & \sum_{i=1}^{p} x_i^2 \end{bmatrix} \begin{bmatrix} w_0 \\ w_1 \end{bmatrix} = \begin{bmatrix} \sum_{i=1}^{p} y_i \\ \sum_{i=1}^{p} y_i x_i \end{bmatrix}. \tag{4.13}$$

Finally, multiplying both sides by the inverse of the square matrix in (4.13) gives the optimal values for w_0 and w_1 as

$$\begin{bmatrix} w_0 \\ w_1 \end{bmatrix} = \begin{bmatrix} p & \sum_{i=1}^{p} x_i \\ \sum_{i=1}^{p} x_i & \sum_{i=1}^{p} x_i^2 \end{bmatrix}^{-1} \begin{bmatrix} \sum_{i=1}^{p} y_i \\ \sum_{i=1}^{p} y_i x_i \end{bmatrix}. \tag{4.14}$$

Example 4.1 (Training a Linear Regressor) Here, we use the least squares solution derived in (4.14) to find the best fitting line for the noisy dataset shown in Fig. 4.2, where

$$\begin{aligned}(x_1, y_1) &= (0, -2),\\(x_2, y_2) &= (2, 1),\\(x_3, y_3) &= (4, 0.5),\\(x_4, y_4) &= (6, 4).\end{aligned} \tag{4.15}$$

Substituting

$$\sum_{i=1}^{4} x_i = 12, \quad \sum_{i=1}^{4} x_i^2 = 56, \quad \sum_{i=1}^{4} y_i = 3.5, \quad \sum_{i=1}^{4} y_i x_i = 28, \tag{4.16}$$

into (4.14) yields

$$\begin{bmatrix} w_0 \\ w_1 \end{bmatrix} = \begin{bmatrix} 4 & 12 \\ 12 & 56 \end{bmatrix}^{-1} \begin{bmatrix} 3.5 \\ 28 \end{bmatrix} = \begin{bmatrix} -1.75 \\ 0.875 \end{bmatrix}. \tag{4.17}$$

Therefore, $f(x) = -1.75 + 0.875\,x$ is the best linear function to represent the dataset in (4.15).

Linear Regression with Multi-Dimensional Input

Up to this point in the chapter, the inputs we dealt with were all scalars or one-dimensional, which allowed us to visualize them as we did in Figs. 4.1 and 4.2. In general, however, the input to regression problems can be, and often, multi-dimensional. While we cannot visualize datasets wherein the input has more than two components or dimensions, nonetheless the least squares framework can be carried over with minimal adjustments to deal with multi-dimensional input.

First, we must expand the linear function definition to accommodate general n-dimensional inputs. Analogously to (4.3), a linear function in n dimensions is defined as

$$f(x_1, x_2, \ldots, x_n) = w_0 + w_1x_1 + w_2x_2 + \cdots + w_nx_n, \tag{4.18}$$

where w_0 is (still) the *bias* parameter, and each input x_i is multiplied by a corresponding *slope* parameter w_i for all $i = 1, 2, \ldots, n$. In a similar manner to what was discussed in Sect. "The Least Squares Cost Function" and shown in (4.9), the least squares cost function for n-dimensional input can be derived as

$$g(w_0, w_1, \ldots, w_n) = \frac{1}{p} \sum_{i=1}^{p} (w_0 + w_1 x_i + \cdots + w_n x_n - y_i)^2. \tag{4.19}$$

At this point, it is notationally convenient to throw all the inputs x_1 through x_n into a single *input* vector denoted as

$$\mathbf{x} = \begin{bmatrix} x_1 \\ x_2 \\ \vdots \\ x_n \end{bmatrix}, \tag{4.20}$$

and all the slope parameters w_1 through w_n into a single *weight* vector denoted as

$$\mathbf{w} = \begin{bmatrix} w_1 \\ w_2 \\ \vdots \\ w_n \end{bmatrix}, \tag{4.21}$$

so that the least squares cost function in (4.19) can be written more compactly as

$$g(w_0, \mathbf{w}) = \frac{1}{p} \sum_{i=1}^{p} (w_0 + \mathbf{w}^T \mathbf{x}_i - y_i)^2. \tag{4.22}$$

Next, we find the partial derivative of $g(\cdot)$ with respect to w_0

$$\frac{\partial g}{\partial w_0} = \frac{1}{p} \sum_{i=1}^{p} 2\,(w_0 + \mathbf{w}^T \mathbf{x}_i - y_i) \frac{\partial (w_0 + \mathbf{w}^T \mathbf{x}_i - y_i)}{\partial w_0} = \frac{2}{p} \sum_{i=1}^{p} (w_0 + \mathbf{w}^T \mathbf{x}_i - y_i) \tag{4.23}$$

and set it to 0, which yields (after simple rearrangements)

$$p\, w_0 + \left(\sum_{i=1}^{p} \mathbf{x}_i^T \right) \mathbf{w} = \sum_{i=1}^{p} y_i. \tag{4.24}$$

Since $\mathbf{w}$ is an $n \times 1$ vector, we must find the *gradient* of $g(\cdot)$ with respect to $\mathbf{w}$

$$\nabla_{\mathbf{w}}\, g = \frac{1}{p}\sum_{i=1}^{p} 2\,(w_0 + \mathbf{w}^T\mathbf{x}_i - y_i)\nabla_{\mathbf{w}}(w_0 + \mathbf{w}^T\mathbf{x}_i - y_i) = \frac{2}{p}\sum_{i=1}^{p}(w_0 + \mathbf{w}^T\mathbf{x}_i - y_i)\mathbf{x}_i \tag{4.25}$$

and set it to $\mathbf{0}_{n\times 1}$. Again, after a few simple rearrangements, we have

$$\left(\sum_{i=1}^{p}\mathbf{x}_i\right) w_0 + \left(\sum_{i=1}^{p}\mathbf{x}_i\mathbf{x}_i^T\right)\mathbf{w} = \sum_{i=1}^{p} y_i\mathbf{x}_i. \tag{4.26}$$

Defining the $(n+1)\times(n+1)$ square matrix $\mathbf{A}$ as

$$\mathbf{A} = \begin{bmatrix} p & \sum_{i=1}^{p}\mathbf{x}_i^T \\ \sum_{i=1}^{p}\mathbf{x}_i & \sum_{i=1}^{p}\mathbf{x}_i\mathbf{x}_i^T \end{bmatrix}, \tag{4.27}$$

and the $(n+1)\times 1$ column vector $\mathbf{b}$ as

$$\mathbf{b} = \begin{bmatrix} \sum_{i=1}^{p} y_i \\ \sum_{i=1}^{p} y_i\mathbf{x}_i \end{bmatrix}, \tag{4.28}$$

we can combine (4.24) and (4.26) into the following linear system of equations:

$$\mathbf{A}\begin{bmatrix} w_0 \\ \mathbf{w} \end{bmatrix} = \mathbf{b}, \tag{4.29}$$

whose solution reveals the optimal values for the parameters of the linear function in (4.18), as

$$\begin{bmatrix} w_0 \\ \mathbf{w} \end{bmatrix} = \mathbf{A}^{-1}\mathbf{b}. \tag{4.30}$$

Example 4.2 (Prediction of Life Expectancy) The Global Health Observatory is a public data repository maintained by the World Health Organization (WHO) and contains various health-related statistics from more than 190 countries across the world. These health-related statistics include adult, children, and infant mortality rates, immunization information, prevalence of certain infectious diseases, and so forth.

(continued)

Example 4.2 (continued)
Here, we show a small slice of this dataset in Table 4.1 that we will use to train a linear regression model for predicting life expectancy based on three input factors including: (i) the adult mortality rate per 1000 population ("Mortality rate"), (ii) the percentage of infants immunized against Polio ("Polio immunization"), and (iii) the per capita gross domestic product reported in U.S. dollars ("GDP"). The output ("Life expectancy") is measured in years. We use the top half of the data shown in Table 4.1 (i.e., the countries whose names start with the letter "A") for training purposes and the bottom half (i.e., the countries whose names start with the letter "B") for validation.
Focusing on the top half of the data, we can compute the matrix **A** in (4.27) as

$$\mathbf{A} = \begin{bmatrix} 9 & 1245.5 & 745.2 & 90265.6 \\ 1245.5 & 263018.6 & 92854.8 & 7402681.9 \\ 745.2 & 92854.8 & 63700.6 & 7963111.5 \\ 90265.6 & 7402681.9 & 7963111.5 & 2445298875.4 \end{bmatrix} \tag{4.31}$$

and the vector **b** in (4.28) as

(continued)

Table 4.1 The dataset associated with Example 4.2. See text for details

	Inputs			Output
Country	Mortality rate	Polio immunization (%)	GDP	Life expectancy
Afghanistan	269.06	48.38	340.02	58.19
Albania	45.06	98.13	2119.73	75.16
Algeria	102.82	93.18	3261.29	74.21
Angola	362.75	70.88	2935.76	50.68
Argentina	100.38	94.46	6932.55	75.24
Armenia	117.33	88.67	2108.68	73.31
Australia	62.43	91.86	35, 391.20	81.91
Austria	65.80	85.53	33, 171.58	81.48
Azerbaijan	119.85	74.08	4004.78	71.15
Bangladesh	135.67	87.67	573.58	69.97
Belarus	220.27	89.27	3669.02	69.75
Belgium	69.93	97.67	17, 752.53	80.65
Belize	154.20	95.60	3871.88	69.15
Benin	269.31	65.38	572.45	57.71
Bhutan	231.53	88.80	1270.01	65.92
Bosnia	63.55	75.18	2216.64	76.18
Brazil	151.27	98.33	5968.89	73.27
Bulgaria	124.73	94.47	4802.02	72.74

Example 4.2 (continued)

$$\mathbf{b} = \begin{bmatrix} 641.3 \\ 80212.3 \\ 54066.7 \\ 7132595.6 \end{bmatrix} \tag{4.32}$$

to calculate the model parameters as

$$\begin{bmatrix} w_0 \\ w_1 \\ w_2 \\ w_3 \end{bmatrix} = \mathbf{A}^{-1}\mathbf{b} = \begin{bmatrix} 79.0 \\ -0.08174 \\ 0.02152 \\ 0.00018 \end{bmatrix}. \tag{4.33}$$

With these retrieved parameters, the final linear model of life expectancy can be written as

$$\begin{aligned} \text{Life expectancy} = 79.0 &- (0.08174 \times \text{Mortality rate}) \\ &+ (0.02152 \times \text{Polio immunization}) \\ &+ (0.00018 \times \text{GDP}). \end{aligned} \tag{4.34}$$

We can now use this model to predict life expectancy for countries in the validation set starting with Bangladesh, which according to Table 4.1 has a mortality rate of 135.67 per 1000 population, an infant Polio immunization rate of 87.67%, and a per capita GDP of 573.58 dollars. Plugging these values into the linear regression model in (4.34), we can find the predicted life expectancy as

$$79.0 - (0.08174 \times 135.6) + (0.02152 \times 87.67) + (0.00018 \times 573.58) = 69.91, \tag{4.35}$$

which is extremely close to the actual life expectancy of 69.97 years in Bangladesh. The same process can be repeated for all countries in the validation set (see Fig. 4.3). Finally, the mean squared error for the validation set can be found, using (4.9), as

$$\text{MSE} = 7.79. \tag{4.36}$$

Input Normalization

The weights or parameters of a linear regression model carry valuable information about the relationship between the input and output data. We saw in (4.34) how life expectancy (output) can be connected linearly to three input factors including

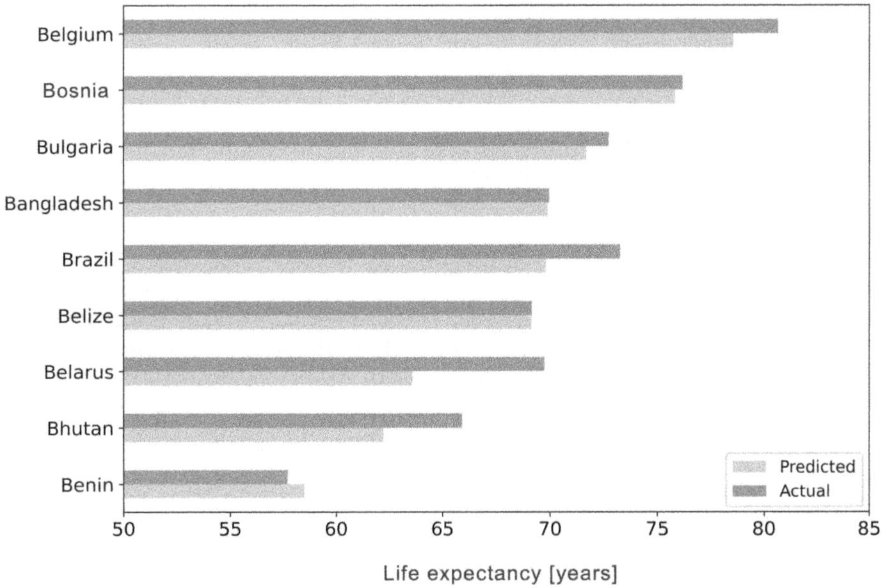

Fig. 4.3 The visual comparison of predicted versus actual life expectancy values for countries whose names start with the letter "B." The actual life expectancy values (in blue) were taken from the dataset in Table 4.1, whereas the predicted values (in yellow) were obtained using the linear regression model in (4.34). It is important to emphasize that the data for the countries shown in this figure were not used during training

mortality rate, Polio immunization, and GDP. The weight associated with mortality rate in this model is negative. This means that decreasing mortality rate would increase life expectancy. On the other hand, the weights associated with the other two inputs are positive, meaning that increasing Polio immunization and GDP would increase life expectancy. In other words, the mathematical *sign* of a particular parameter in a linear regression model determines whether the input attached to that parameter contributes negatively or positively to the output.

The *magnitude* of a parameter also informs us about how strongly the output is correlated with the input associated with that parameter. Intuitively, the larger the input's weight the greater its influence on the output. This insight can be used to create a ranking of the inputs' importance based on their contribution to the output. However, there is one caveat: when $|w_i| > |w_j|$, we may conclude that the ith input has a greater effect than the jth input, *only if* the two inputs are on a comparable scale.

For example, from (4.34), it is not immediately clear that Polio immunization has a larger influence on determining life expectancy than GDP just because the weight associated with Polio immunization (i.e., 0.02152) is greater in magnitude than the weight associated with GDP (i.e., 0.00018). This is because Polio immunization (as a percentage) always ranges between 0 and 100, whereas the per capita GDP can vary from a few hundred dollars in developing countries to tens of thousands of dollars in certain developed countries (see Table 4.1).

Luckily, this lack of harmony is something we can fix via *input normalization*. Suppose that the input x_i in a regression dataset ranges from a_i to b_i, i.e., $a_i \leq x_i \leq b_i$. By subtracting a_i from x_i and dividing the result by $b_i - a_i$, we can define a linearly scaled version of x_i denoted as

$$x_i' = \frac{x_i - a_i}{b_i - a_i}, \qquad i = 1, 2, \ldots, p. \tag{4.37}$$

This simple input normalization scheme is precisely what we want as it ensures that x_i' always lies between 0 and 1 (see Exercise 4.3). Moreover, it does not invalidate any of our previous modeling assumptions, since, from a mathematical standpoint, a linear function with tunable parameters involving x_i''s as input is equivalent to one involving x_i's as input. Recall from (4.18) that a linear model having $x_1', x_2', \ldots, x_n'$ as input can be written as

$$\begin{aligned}
f(x_1', x_2', \ldots, x_n') &= w_0 + \sum_{i=1}^{n} w_i\, x_i' \\
&= w_0 + \sum_{i=1}^{n} w_i \left(\frac{x_i - a_i}{b_i - a_i}\right) \\
&= \underbrace{w_0 - \sum_{i=1}^{n} \frac{w_i\, a_i}{b_i - a_i}}_{v_0} + \sum_{i=1}^{n} \underbrace{\frac{w_i}{b_i - a_i}}_{v_i} x_i \\
&= v_0 + \sum_{i=1}^{n} v_i\, x_i,
\end{aligned} \tag{4.38}$$

which remains a linear function in $x_1, x_2, \ldots, x_n$, albeit with a different set of parameters (v_0 through v_n).

Example 4.3 (Revisiting Prediction of Life Expectancy) Here, we repeat the steps taken in Example 4.2 to create a linear regression model of life expectancy. This time, we normalize the input data first so that we can use the resulting least squares solution to compare the relative importance of each input in estimating the output.

For each input column in Table 4.1, we find the smallest and largest values across all countries, denoting them as a and b, respectively. We then use the linear transformation $x \mapsto \frac{x-a}{b-a}$ to form the normalized dataset shown in Table 4.2. Note that the normalization procedure must be performed over the whole dataset that includes both the training and validation subsets of the data.

(continued)

Table 4.2 The dataset associated with Example 4.3. See text for details

	Normalized inputs			Output
Country	Mortality rate	Polio immunization	GDP	Life expectancy
Afghanistan	0.70510	0.0000	0.0000	58.19
Albania	0.0000	0.9958	0.05078	75.16
Algeria	0.1818	0.8969	0.0833	74.21
Angola	1.0000	0.4504	0.0741	50.68
Argentina	0.1741	0.9225	0.1881	75.24
Armenia	0.2275	0.8065	0.0505	73.31
Australia	0.0547	0.8704	1.0000	81.91
Austria	0.0653	0.7438	0.9367	81.48
Azerbaijan	0.2354	0.5145	0.1046	71.15
Bangladesh	0.2852	0.7865	0.0067	69.97
Belarus	0.5515	0.8185	0.0950	69.75
Belgium	0.0783	0.9867	0.4968	80.65
Belize	0.3435	0.9453	0.1008	69.15
Benin	0.7059	0.3405	0.0066	57.71
Bhutan	0.5870	0.8092	0.0265	65.92
Bosnia	0.0582	0.5366	0.0535	76.18
Brazil	0.3343	1.0000	0.1606	73.27
Bulgaria	0.2508	0.9226	0.1273	72.74

Example 4.3 (continued)

Following (4.30), the least squares solution can be calculated as

$$\begin{bmatrix} w_0 \\ w_1 \\ w_2 \\ w_3 \end{bmatrix} = \begin{bmatrix} 9.0000 & 2.6439 & 6.2007 & 2.4879 \\ 2.6439 & 1.6749 & 1.1748 & 0.2739 \\ 6.2007 & 1.1748 & 5.0758 & 1.9937 \\ 2.4879 & 0.2739 & 1.9937 & 1.9412 \end{bmatrix}^{-1} \begin{bmatrix} 641.31 \\ 161.52 \\ 461.25 \\ 197.27 \end{bmatrix} = \begin{bmatrix} 76.42 \\ -25.97 \\ 1.08 \\ 6.24 \end{bmatrix}. \tag{4.39}$$

Using these parameters, the linear model in (4.34) can be rewritten as

$$\begin{aligned} \text{Life expectancy} = 76.42 &- (25.97 \times \text{Mortality rate}) \\ &+ (1.08 \times \text{Polio immunization}) \\ &+ (6.24 \times \text{GDP}), \end{aligned} \tag{4.40}$$

where the magnitude of the weight of each input can now be used as a proxy for determining the extent of its contribution toward estimating the output. In this example, the weight attached to mortality rate has the largest magnitude followed by GDP and Polio immunization.

Regularization

In all regression problems, we have discussed so far the number of data points p always exceeded the number of inputs n. In this section, we discuss what happens when the reverse is true, i.e., $n \geq p$. As done previously, we start with a simple toy dataset with $n = p = 2$

$$\begin{aligned} (x_{1,1},\ x_{1,2},\ y_1) &= (0,\ 0,\ 1), \\ (x_{2,1},\ x_{2,2},\ y_2) &= (1,\ 1,\ 2), \end{aligned} \tag{4.41}$$

in order to flesh out the important ideas involved.

Leveraging the linear function $f(x_1, x_2) = w_0 + w_1 x_1 + w_2 x_2$, we can form the following linear system of equations:

$$\begin{aligned} w_0 \qquad\qquad &= 1, \\ w_0 + w_1 + w_2 &= 2, \end{aligned} \tag{4.42}$$

to model the data in (4.41). It quickly becomes clear that this system has many solutions. More precisely, any set of parameters of the form $(w_0, w_1, w_2) = (1, t, 1-t)$ is a solution to (4.42), where t can be any real number. For example, $t = 1, t = 10$, and $t = 100$ yield the linear functions $1 + x_1$, $1 + 10x_1 - 9x_2$, and $1 + 100x_1 - 90x_2$, respectively, all of which can explain the data in (4.41) perfectly and without error.

When $n \geq p$, the resulting linear system of equations, like the one shown in (4.42), has fewer equations than unknowns, which leads to the possibility of it having infinitely many solutions. This results in the least squares cost function

$$g(w_0, w_1, w_2) = \frac{1}{2}\sum_{i=1}^{2}(w_0 + w_1 x_{i,1} + w_2 x_{i,2} - y_i)^2 \tag{4.43}$$

to have infinitely many minima, which, practically speaking, is not desirable. One way to address this issue is to adjust the least squares cost function by adding a non-negative function $r(w_1, w_2)$ to the original cost

$$g(w_0, w_1, w_2) + r(w_1, w_2) \tag{4.44}$$

so that the new cost function has a unique minimum. The function $r(\cdot)$ is called a *regularizer*, and the adjustment process described above is referred to as *regularization*. The most commonly used regularizer in deep learning is the *quadratic* or *ridge* regularizer defined as

$$r(w_1, w_2) = \lambda \left(w_1^2 + w_2^2\right), \tag{4.45}$$

where $\lambda \geq 0$ is a tunable parameter commonly referred to as the *regularization parameter*. When it comes to minimizing the regularized least squares cost in (4.44), notice how the existence of the regularization function discourages both w_1 and w_2 from attaining very large values. When $\lambda = 0$, the regularized cost reduces to the original least squares cost in (4.43). Conversely, when λ is set fairly large, the regularizer function dominates the original cost, pushing w_1 and w_2 toward zero in the cost function's minimum. In practice, the regularization parameter λ can be set to a small value, particularly when the input data is normalized (as discussed in the previous section).

Writing the regularized least squares cost function in (4.44), using general n and p, as

$$\frac{1}{p}\sum_{i=1}^{p}(w_0 + \mathbf{w}^T\mathbf{x}_i - y_i)^2 + \lambda\, \mathbf{w}^T\mathbf{w}, \tag{4.46}$$

we can follow the steps laid down in (4.23) through (4.30) to find the least squares solution as

$$\begin{bmatrix} w_0 \\ \\ \mathbf{w} \end{bmatrix} = \mathbf{A}^{-1}\mathbf{b}, \tag{4.47}$$

where

$$\mathbf{A} = \begin{bmatrix} p & \sum_{i=1}^{p}\mathbf{x}_i^T \\ \\ \sum_{i=1}^{p}\mathbf{x}_i & \left(\sum_{i=1}^{p}\mathbf{x}_i\mathbf{x}_i^T\right) + \lambda\, \mathbf{I}_{n\times n} \end{bmatrix}, \qquad \mathbf{b} = \begin{bmatrix} \sum_{i=1}^{p} y_i \\ \\ \sum_{i=1}^{p} y_i\mathbf{x}_i \end{bmatrix}, \tag{4.48}$$

and where $\mathbf{I}_{n\times n}$ is the identity matrix.

Example 4.4 (Regularized Linear Regression) Here, we train a linear regression model for the toy dataset in (4.41) using the regularized least squares solution derived in (4.47). Substituting

$$p = 2, \quad \mathbf{x}_1 = \begin{bmatrix} 0 \\ 0 \end{bmatrix}, \quad \mathbf{x}_2 = \begin{bmatrix} 1 \\ 1 \end{bmatrix}, \quad y_1 = 1, \quad y_2 = 2, \tag{4.49}$$

into (4.48), we have

$$\begin{bmatrix} w_0 \\ w_1 \\ w_2 \end{bmatrix} = \begin{bmatrix} 2 & 1 & 1 \\ 1 & 1+\lambda & 1 \\ 1 & 1 & 1+\lambda \end{bmatrix}^{-1} \begin{bmatrix} 3 \\ 2 \\ 2 \end{bmatrix}. \tag{4.50}$$

(continued)

Example 4.4 (continued)
Note that when $\lambda = 0$, the square matrix $\mathbf{A}$ in (4.50) is not invertible. This is indeed the reason why we regularize the least squares cost function in the first place. However, when $\lambda > 0$, the matrix $\mathbf{A}$ becomes invertible regardless of how small or large λ is. Typically, λ is set fairly small so that the regularization function $r(\cdot)$ does not drown out the original least squares function $g(\cdot)$ in (4.44). For example, setting $\lambda = 0.001$ in (4.50) gives

$$\begin{bmatrix} w_0 \\ w_1 \\ w_2 \end{bmatrix} = \begin{bmatrix} 2 & 1 & 1 \\ 1 & 1.001 & 1 \\ 1 & 1 & 1.001 \end{bmatrix}^{-1} \begin{bmatrix} 3 \\ 2 \\ 2 \end{bmatrix} = \begin{bmatrix} 1.0 \\ 0.5 \\ 0.5 \end{bmatrix}. \tag{4.51}$$

More generally, adding the term $\lambda\, \mathbf{I}_{n\times n}$ inside the matrix $\mathbf{A}$ in (4.48) guarantees $\mathbf{A}$ to be invertible (see Exercise 4.2).

Problems

4.1 Linearity, Additivity, and Homogeneity

(a) A function f is said to be additive if $f(x_1 + x_2) = f(x_1) + f(x_2)$ for every pair of inputs x_1 and x_2. Are all linear functions as defined in (4.3) additive? If not, can you find a sub-family of linear functions that always satisfy the *additivity* property?

(b) A function f is said to be homogeneous if $f(\alpha x) = \alpha f(x)$ for every scalar α. Are all linear functions as defined in (4.3) homogeneous? If not, can you find a sub-family of linear functions that always satisfy the *homogeneity* property?

(c) Show that if a function f is both additive and homogeneous, then we can write $f(\alpha_1 x_1 + \alpha_2 x_2 + \cdots + \alpha_N x_N) = \alpha_1 f(x_1) + \alpha_2 f(x_2) + \cdots + \alpha_N f(x_N)$, where $\alpha_1, \alpha_2, \ldots, \alpha_N$ and $x_1, x_2, \ldots, x_N$ are a set of N arbitrary scalars and inputs, respectively.

4.2 The Least Squares Solution

(a) Show that when $n = 1$, the least squares solution provided for general n-dimensional input in (4.30) reduces to the solution derived in (4.14).

(b) Show that the least squares solution in (4.30) can be written equivalently as

$$\begin{bmatrix} w_0 \\ \\ \mathbf{w} \end{bmatrix} = \left(\mathbf{X}\mathbf{X}^T\right)^{-1} \mathbf{X}\mathbf{y}, \tag{4.52}$$

where the vector $\mathbf{y}$ is formed by throwing all outputs into a single vector

$$\mathbf{y}_{p\times 1} = \begin{bmatrix} y_1 \\ y_2 \\ \vdots \\ y_p \end{bmatrix} \tag{4.53}$$

and where the matrix $\mathbf{X}$ is formed by stacking all input vectors $\mathbf{x}_1$ through $\mathbf{x}_p$ side-by-side as columns of a new matrix, and then extending its row space by adding a row vector consisting only of 1's, as in

$$\mathbf{X}_{(n+1)\times p} = \begin{bmatrix} 1 & 1 & \cdots & 1 \\ \mathbf{x}_1 & \mathbf{x}_2 & \cdots & \mathbf{x}_p \end{bmatrix}. \tag{4.54}$$

(c) Follow a similar set of steps as described in (4.23) through (4.30) to derive (4.47) as the optimal set of parameters that minimize the regularized least squares function in (4.46).

(d) Show that when the least squares cost function is regularized via $r(\mathbf{w}) = \lambda \mathbf{w}^T \mathbf{w}$, the least squares solution in (4.52) can be adjusted and written as

$$\begin{bmatrix} w_0 \\ \\ \mathbf{w} \end{bmatrix} = \left(\mathbf{X}\mathbf{X}^T + \lambda \mathring{\mathbf{I}}\right)^{-1} \mathbf{X}\mathbf{y}, \tag{4.55}$$

where $\mathring{\mathbf{I}}$ is an $(n+1) \times (n+1)$ identity matrix whose first diagonal entry is set to 0.

$$\mathring{\mathbf{I}} = \begin{bmatrix} 0 & 0 & 0 & \cdots & 0 \\ 0 & 1 & 0 & \cdots & 0 \\ 0 & 0 & 1 & \cdots & 0 \\ \vdots & \vdots & \vdots & \ddots & \vdots \\ 0 & 0 & 0 & \cdots & 1 \end{bmatrix}. \tag{4.56}$$

(e) Show that, when $\lambda > 0$, the matrix $\mathbf{X}\mathbf{X}^T + \lambda \mathring{\mathbf{I}}$ in (4.55) is always invertible regardless of the dimensions or entries of $\mathbf{X}$.

4.3 Input Normalization

(a) Given two real numbers c and d (where $c < d$) and a set of p measurements $\{x_1, x_2, \ldots, x_p\}$, find a linear function $f(\cdot)$ such that $c \leq f(x_i) \leq d$ for all $i = 1, 2, \ldots, p$.

(b) Recall from our discussion of input normalization in Sect. "Input Normalization" that the linear model of life expectancy that was originally derived in (4.34) could not be used to infer relative input importance. To remedy this issue, in Example 4.3, we linearly transformed all inputs as shown in Table 4.2 and applied the least squares solution to this normalized data to derive a new linear model in (4.40), in which the input weights *can* be used to infer relative input importance. In this part of the exercise, you will re-derive the linear model in (4.40) without using the normalized data in Table 4.2, but instead by only leveraging (4.38) along with the original (unnormalized) data in Table 4.1.

4.4 Prediction of Life Expectancy: Part I

In Example 4.2, we used a relatively small dataset consisting of $p = 18$ countries to predict life expectancy based on $n = 3$ input factors including mortality rate, Polio immunization rate, and GDP. Here, we use an expanded version of this dataset that contains $p = 133$ countries. This version of the data is stored in `life-expectancy-133-countries.csv` that is included in the chapter's supplements. The goal of this exercise is to evaluate how increasing the *size of data* impacts the prediction power of linear regression, as measured over a validation dataset using the mean squared error (MSE) metric defined in (4.8):

(a) Normalize the input data as described in Sect. "Input Normalization".
(b) Use the normalized data associated with all countries whose names start with the letters "A-M" to train a linear regression model for life expectancy.
(c) Based on your model, which input happens to be the most important factor in predicting the output? Which input happens to be the least important?
(d) Use your trained model to calculate the mean squared error (MSE) for the validation portion of the data that includes all countries whose names start with the letters "N-Z." How does this MSE value compare to the MSE value calculated for the smaller version of the dataset in Table 4.2?

4.5 Prediction of Life Expectancy: Part II

In this exercise, we use an expanded version of the dataset referenced in Exercise 4.4 (with $n = 18$ input factors) to train a linear regression model for predicting life expectancy. This version of the data is stored in `life-expectancy-18-factors.csv` that is included in the chapter's supplements. The goal of this exercise is to evaluate how increasing the *input dimension* impacts the prediction power of linear regression, as measured over a validation dataset using the mean squared error (MSE) metric defined in (4.8):

(a) Normalize the input data as described in Sect. "Input Normalization".
(b) Use the normalized data associated with all countries whose names start with the letters "A-M" to train a linear regression model for life expectancy.
(c) Based on your model, which input happens to be the most important factor in predicting the output? Which input happens to be the least important?
(d) Use your trained model to calculate the mean squared error (MSE) for the validation portion of the data that includes all countries whose names start with the letters "N-Z." How does this MSE value compare to the MSE values calculated for the other smaller versions of this data in Example 4.2 and in Exercise 4.4?

4.6 Prediction of Medical Insurance Costs

In this exercise, we utilize certain demographic and medical information (inputs) to train a linear regression model for prediction of medical insurance charges (output). The input factors include age, body mass index (BMI), the number of children, and smoking status (1 for smokers and 0 for non-smokers). The dataset used here is an abridged version of the "insurance" dataset taken from [1], which is included in the chapter's supplements (under the name `medical-insurance.csv`):

(a) Normalize the input data as described in Sect. "Input Normalization".
(b) Split the data randomly into two equal-sized training and validation datasets, and use the former to train a linear regression model.
(c) Based on your model, which input happens to be the most important factor in predicting the output? Which input happens to be the least important?
(d) Use your trained model to calculate the mean squared error (MSE) for both the training and validation datasets. Which MSE value is larger in this case? Is that what you expected? Explain.

Reference

1. Lantz B. Machine learning with R. Birmingham: Packt Publishing; 2013

Chapter 5
Linear Classification

In the previous chapter, we studied linear regression as the most fundamental model for capturing the relationship between input and output data in situations where output takes on values from a continuous range. Analogously, linear classification is considered to be the foundational classification model for separating two (or more) classes of data using linear boundaries.

Since both paradigms use linear models at their core, our overall treatment of linear classification in this chapter will closely mirror our discussion of linear regression in Chap. 4. However, as we will see shortly, the seemingly subtle distinction between regression and classification (in terms of the nature of the output) leads to significant differences in the cost functions used in each case, as well as the optimization strategies employed to minimize those costs to retrieve optimal model parameters.

Linear Classification with One-Dimensional Input

We begin the chapter, like we did in Sect. "Linear Regression with One-Dimensional Input", by considering a simulated classification dataset consisting only of $p = 6$ input–output pairs of the form (x_i, y_i)

$$\begin{array}{c} (-2.0, 0), \\ (-1.5, 0), \\ (-1.0, 0), \\ (-0.5, 1), \\ (0.5, 1), \\ (2.5, 1), \end{array} \tag{5.1}$$

R. Borhani et al., *Fundamentals of Machine Learning and Deep Learning in Medicine*, https://doi.org/10.1007/978-3-031-19502-0_5

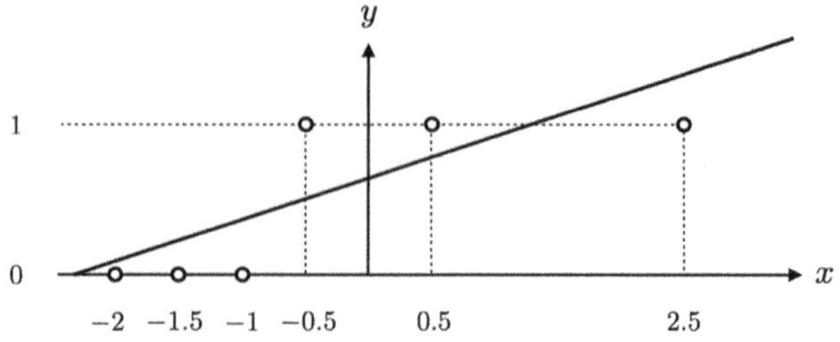

Fig. 5.1 The plot of the simulated classification dataset in (5.1) along with the best linear regressor to fit this data. A regression line is clearly a poor model for representing classification data

where x_i and y_i represent the ith input and output, respectively. As with regression, the goal with classification is to find a function $f(\cdot)$ such that $f(x_i) = y_i$ holds true for $i = 1, 2, \ldots, 6$. Note that because the output y_i is always limited to take on binary values (i.e., 0 or 1), classification can be thought of as a special case of regression (where a special type of constraint is imposed on the values that the output can attain). It is, therefore, not illogical to wonder whether we can reuse the same mathematical framework we developed in the previous chapter to find $f(\cdot)$ in this case as well. Let us give it a try!

Following the same set of steps as outlined in Example 4.1, one can derive the function $f(x) = 0.5875+0.2625\,x$ as the best linear regressor to fit the classification data in (5.1), both of which (the function and the data) are plotted in Fig. 5.1. A quick glance at this figure shows that $f(\cdot)$, having an unconstrained and unbounded output, represents the underlying dataset rather poorly.

This issue can be fixed by employing the so-called Heaviside step function $h(\cdot)$, which is defined as

$$h(x) = \begin{cases} 0, & x < 0 \\ 1, & x \geq 0 \end{cases} \tag{5.2}$$

and plotted in the left panel of Fig. 5.2. Since the output of $h(\cdot)$ is binary at all times, it possesses the properties we expect to see in a proper classification function. Therefore, we can pass the linear function $f(x) = w_0 + w_1 x$ through $h(\cdot)$ and use the compositional function $h(f(x))$ as our new classifier.

A corresponding least squares cost function can be formed, following the steps described in Sect. "The Least Squares Cost Function", as

$$g(w_0, w_1) = \frac{1}{p}\sum_{i=1}^{p}(h(f(x_i)) - y_i)^2 = \frac{1}{p}\sum_{i=1}^{p}(h(w_0 + w_1 x_i) - y_i)^2, \tag{5.3}$$

which closely resembles the least squares cost function in (4.9). This time, however, we cannot simply set the partial derivatives of $g(\cdot)$ to zero and solve for w_0 and

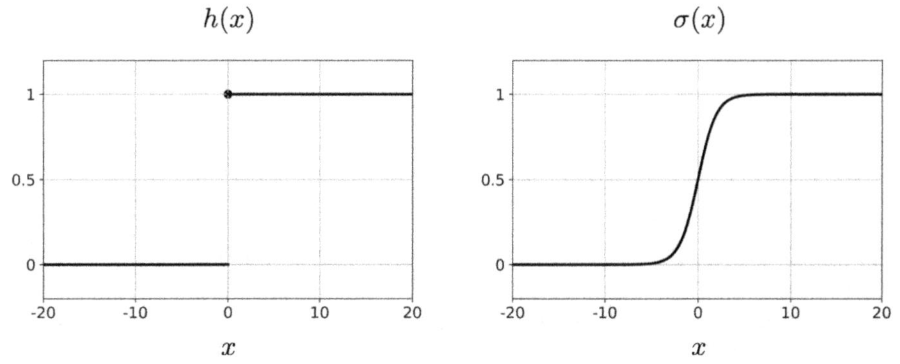

Fig. 5.2 (Left panel) The Heaviside step function defined in (5.2). (Right panel) The logistic function defined in (5.4). In practice, the logistic function can be used as a smooth and differentiable approximation to the Heaviside step function

w_1, since the function $h(\cdot)$ contained within $g(\cdot)$ is discontinuous and hence non-differentiable.[1]

A clever way to get around this issue is to replace $h(\cdot)$ with another function approximating it that is smooth and differentiable. The logistic function defined as

$$\sigma(x) = \frac{1}{1 + e^{-x}} \tag{5.4}$$

and plotted in the right panel of Fig. 5.2 is one such function. In the next section, we will take a closer look at this function, its historical origins, and its mathematical properties.

The Logistic Function

The first recorded use of the logistic function dates back to the mid-nineteenth century and the work of the Belgian mathematician Pierre Francois Verhulst who used this function in his study of population growth. Prior to Verhulst, the Malthusian model was the only game in town when it came to modeling how biological populations grew over time. The Malthusian model assumes that the rate of growth in a population at each point in time is proportional to the size of the

[1] Technically, it is feasible to use *subderivatives* and *subgradients* [1] to bypass the issue of non-differentiability of the Heaviside function. However, as we will see later in the chapter, there are additional reasons making the least squares cost function in (5.3) inappropriate for use in classification problems.

population at that point. Expressed mathematically, the Malthusian model assumes that

$$\frac{\mathrm{d}}{\mathrm{d}t}N(t) \propto N(t), \tag{5.5}$$

where $N(t)$ denotes the size of the population at time t and the $\propto$ symbol denotes proportionality.[2] Based on the Malthusian model, as the population gets larger in size so does the rate of the growth of the population, causing $N(t)$ to grow *exponentially* in time. Indeed, one can easily verify that the exponential function $N(t) = e^t$ satisfies (5.5).

The Malthusian model is quite effective in explaining bacterial growth, among many other biological processes. Starting with a single bacterium at time $t = 0$, and assuming that binary fission (i.e., the division of one bacterium into two) takes exactly one second to complete, at $t = 1$ there will be $N = 2$ bacteria, at $t = 2$ there will be $N = 4$ bacteria, at $t = 3$ there will be $N = 8$ bacteria, etc. The question is: can this exponential pattern continue forever?

When the resources needed for the growth of a population (e.g., food, space, etc.) are limited, there comes a point at which the growth begins to slow down. To incorporate this reality into his growth model, Verhulst used an adjusted growth rate of $N(t)(K - N(t))$, wherein the constant K represents the capacity of the system that hosts the population. This way, the growth rate is influenced by not only the population at time t but also by the remaining capacity in the system at time t, via the term $K - N(t)$.

With this adjustment, Verhulst re-wrote the differential equation in (5.5) as

$$\frac{\mathrm{d}}{\mathrm{d}t}N(t) \propto N(t)(K - N(t)) \tag{5.6}$$

and derived the logistic function in (5.4) as a solution (see Fig. 5.3 and Exercise 5.3).

The differential equation in (5.6), commonly referred to as the logistic equation, has found many applications outside its originating field of ecology. In medicine, the logistic equation has been used to model tumor growth in mice and humans [3, 4], where in this context $N(t)$ represents the volume of tumor at time t. In another set of medical applications, the logistic equation has been employed to model the spread of infectious diseases, where in this context $N(t)$ represents the number of cases of the disease at time t. In certain circumstances, $N(t)$ closely follows a logistic pattern, e.g., the SARS outbreak in the beginning of the twenty first century [5], and more recently the Covid-19 pandemic [6]. A clear logistic trend is discernible in Fig. 5.4 that shows the number of Covid-19 cases in China over a 3-month period starting from January 3, 2020 and ending on April 3, 2020.

[2] $f(t) \propto g(t)$ is another way of stating that there always exists a constant α such that $f(t) = \alpha\, g(t)$.

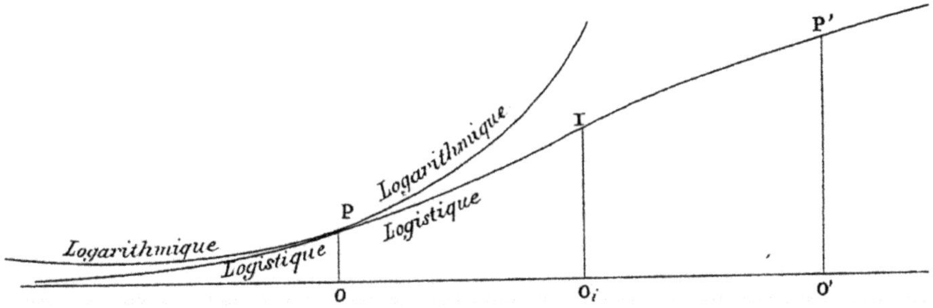

Fig. 5.3 A hand-drawn depiction of the logistic ("Logistique") function in an 1845 paper by Verhulst [2], in which he compares his model of population growth with the exponential ("Logarithmique") model. In Verhulst's sketch of the logistic function, the rate of growth peaks around the point labeled as O_i, and the population curve starts to level off around the point labeled as O'

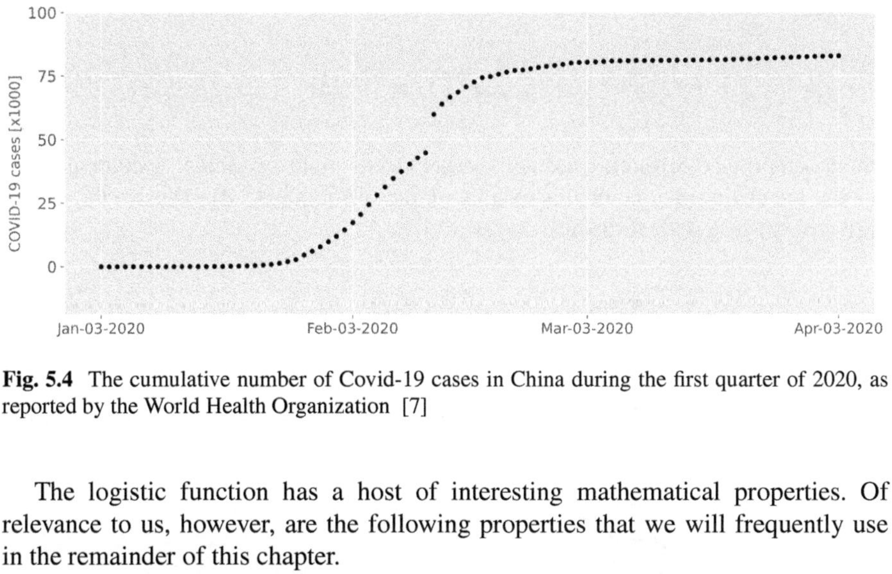

Fig. 5.4 The cumulative number of Covid-19 cases in China during the first quarter of 2020, as reported by the World Health Organization [7]

The logistic function has a host of interesting mathematical properties. Of relevance to us, however, are the following properties that we will frequently use in the remainder of this chapter.

First, the logistic function $\sigma(\cdot)$ is monotonically increasing, meaning that $\sigma(t_1) > \sigma(t_2)$ if and only if $t_1 > t_2$. It always ranges between 0 and 1 and satisfies

$$\sigma(-t) = 1 - \sigma(t). \tag{5.7}$$

The derivative of $\sigma(\cdot)$ can be written in terms of $\sigma(\cdot)$ itself, as

$$\frac{\mathrm{d}}{\mathrm{d}t}\sigma(t) = \sigma(t)\,\sigma(-t) = \sigma(t)\,(1 - \sigma(t)). \tag{5.8}$$

Finally, the logistic function is closely related to the hyperbolic tangent function

$$\tanh(t) = \frac{\sinh(t)}{\cosh(t)} = \frac{\frac{1}{2}\left(e^{t} - e^{-t}\right)}{\frac{1}{2}\left(e^{t} + e^{-t}\right)} = \frac{e^{2t} - 1}{e^{2t} + 1} \tag{5.9}$$

via the identity

$$\sigma(t) = \frac{1 + \tanh\left(\frac{t}{2}\right)}{2}. \tag{5.10}$$

The Cross-Entropy Cost Function

Replacing the Heaviside step function $h(\cdot)$ with the logistic function $\sigma(\cdot)$ in (5.3) gives a new least squares cost of the form

$$g(w_0, w_1) = \frac{1}{p} \sum_{i=1}^{p} \left(\sigma\left(w_0 + w_1 x_i\right) - y_i\right)^2, \tag{5.11}$$

which can now be differentiated with respect to its input variables. Specifically, we can use the chain rule of calculus along with the formula in (5.8) to derive the partial derivative of $g(\cdot)$ with respect to w_0, as

$$\begin{aligned} \frac{\partial g}{\partial w_0} &= \frac{1}{p} \sum_{i=1}^{p} 2\left(\sigma_i - y_i\right) \frac{\partial\left(\sigma_i - y_i\right)}{\partial w_0} \\ &= \frac{2}{p} \sum_{i=1}^{p} \left(\sigma_i - y_i\right) \sigma_i \left(1 - \sigma_i\right) \frac{\partial\left(w_0 + w_1 x_i\right)}{\partial w_0} \\ &= \frac{2}{p} \sum_{i=1}^{p} \left(\sigma_i - y_i\right) \sigma_i \left(1 - \sigma_i\right), \end{aligned} \tag{5.12}$$

where we have replaced $\sigma\left(w_0 + w_1 x_i\right)$ with σ_i to simplify the notation. Similarly, the partial derivative of $g(\cdot)$ with respect to w_1 can be written, and simplified, as

$$\frac{\partial g}{\partial w_1} = \frac{2}{p} \sum_{i=1}^{p} \left(\sigma_i - y_i\right) \sigma_i \left(1 - \sigma_i\right) x_i. \tag{5.13}$$

Setting both partial derivatives to zero gives the following system of equations:

$$\begin{aligned}
&\sum_{i=1}^{p}\left(\frac{1}{1+e^{-(w_0+w_1x_i)}}-y_i\right)\frac{e^{-(w_0+w_1x_i)}}{\left(1+e^{-(w_0+w_1x_i)}\right)^2}=0,\\
&\sum_{i=1}^{p}\left(\frac{1}{1+e^{-(w_0+w_1x_i)}}-y_i\right)\frac{x_i\,e^{-(w_0+w_1x_i)}}{\left(1+e^{-(w_0+w_1x_i)}\right)^2}=0,
\end{aligned} \tag{5.14}$$

to be solved for w_0 and w_1.

Make sure to take a moment and compare this rather convoluted system of equations with its much simpler regression analog in (4.12). Although we were able to solve the linear system in (4.12) with relative ease, we cannot do the same here due to the nonlinearity injected into (5.14) as a consequence of employing the logistic function. In other words, unlike the linear system in (4.12), the nonlinear system of equations in (5.14) has no known closed-form algebraic solution. This motivates the introduction of a different cost function for linear classification, commonly referred to as the cross-entropy cost, which we derive next.

Using the notation $\sigma_i = \sigma(w_0 + w_1x_i)$, notice how the least squares cost function in (5.11), which can be rewritten as

$$g(w_0, w_1) = \frac{1}{p}\sum_{i=1}^{p}(\sigma_i - y_i)^2, \tag{5.15}$$

incentivizes $\sigma_i \approx y_i$ to hold as tightly as possible. The closer the values of σ_i and y_i, the better the approximation, and the smaller the value of $g(w_0, w_1)$. This was the basis of the least squares cost function derived originally in (4.9). As discussed earlier in the chapter, classification is a special case of regression where y_i's are bound to be either 0 or 1. This unique property of the output can be leveraged to formulate a new cost function specifically tailored to classification problems.

Starting with the case of $y_i = 1$, it is clear that we want σ_i to be as close to 1 as possible. Inverting σ_i, we want $\frac{1}{\sigma_i}$ to be as small as possible (recall that $0 < \sigma_i < 1$). Therefore, $\frac{1}{\sigma_i}$ seems to be an appropriate penalty term for the ith input–output pair to ensure $\sigma_i \approx y_i = 1$. A loose approximation in this case pushes σ_i away from 1 and toward 0, causing the term $\frac{1}{\sigma_i}$ to become exceedingly large.

A similar argument can be made when $y_i = 0$. In this case, we want σ_i to be as close to 0 as possible. Here, $\frac{1}{1-\sigma_i}$ seems to be an appropriate penalty term for the ith input–output pair to ensure $\sigma_i \approx y_i = 0$. Since σ_i always ranges between 0 and 1, a loose approximation in this case pushes σ_i away from 0 and toward 1, causing the term $\frac{1}{1-\sigma_i}$ to explode.

The two cases discussed above (i.e., $y_i = 0$ and $y_i = 1$) can be combined in a clever way into a single mathematical expression defined as

$$g_i = \left(\frac{1}{\sigma_i}\right)^{y_i} \left(\frac{1}{1-\sigma_i}\right)^{1-y_i}. \tag{5.16}$$

Clearly, g_i reduces to $\frac{1}{\sigma_i}$ when $y_i = 1$ and to $\frac{1}{1-\sigma_i}$ when $y_i = 0$. To avoid dealing with gargantuan numbers when σ_i deviates from y_i, we can take the natural logarithm of g_i

$$\log(g_i) = -\left(y_i \log(\sigma_i) + (1-y_i)\log(1-\sigma_i)\right), \tag{5.17}$$

which, by design, converts very large numbers into considerably smaller ones.[3] Finally, taking the average of all the terms in (5.17) across the entire dataset forms the cross-entropy cost function

$$g(w_0, w_1) = -\frac{1}{p}\sum_{i=1}^{p} y_i \log(\sigma_i) + (1-y_i)\log(1-\sigma_i). \tag{5.18}$$

As a *convex* function, the cross-entropy cost in (5.18) has an important practical advantage over its non-convex least squares counterpart in (5.15). Owing to their unique geometry, convex functions are generally much easier to optimize compared to non-convex functions.

Taking a similar set of steps as outlined in the beginning of this section, we can form the nonlinear system of equations (akin to the one shown in (5.14))

$$\begin{aligned} \sum_{i=1}^{p} \frac{1}{1+e^{-(w_0+w_1x_i)}} &= \sum_{i=1}^{p} y_i, \\ \sum_{i=1}^{p} \frac{x_i}{1+e^{-(w_0+w_1x_i)}} &= \sum_{i=1}^{p} y_i\, x_i, \end{aligned} \tag{5.19}$$

and solve it for optimal w_0 and w_1. Although this new system of equations is less complex-looking than the system in (5.14), it still possesses no known algebraic solution that can be written in closed form. This is where optimization algorithms (e.g., gradient descent) must be employed, as we discuss next.

[3] Replacing g_i with its logarithm is permitted because $\log(\cdot)$ is a monotonically increasing function over its domain. If $g_i > g_j$ for some i and j, we will still have $\log(g_i) > \log(g_j)$ after passing each term through the $\log(\cdot)$ function.

The Gradient Descent Algorithm

Up to this point in the book, our method of minimizing a given cost function has involved setting the partial derivatives of the function (with respect to its inputs) to zero and solving the resulting system of equations for optimal input values. This strategy was effective in minimizing the least squares cost functions associated with linear regression in (4.9), (4.22), and (4.46). In each case, the resulting system was linear in its unknown variables, making it easy to solve using basic linear algebra manipulations. Despite the fact that these systems all had a unique solution, this general strategy works even when the derivative system has multiple solutions.

Consider the single input function

$$g(w) = \frac{1}{6}w^6 - \frac{3}{5}w^5 + \frac{1}{4}w^4 + w^3 - w^2 + 2 \tag{5.20}$$

for instance. The derivative of this polynomial function can be computed as

$$\frac{dg}{dw} = w^5 - 3w^4 + w^3 + 3w^2 - 2w = (w-2)(w-1)^2\, w\,(w+1), \tag{5.21}$$

which has multiple zeros at $w = 2$, $w = 1$, $w = 0$, and $w = -1$. The points at which the derivative of a function becomes zero are often referred to as the function's *stationary points*. These may include local minima, local maxima, and saddle (or inflection) points. The plot of $g(\cdot)$ in Fig. 5.5 shows two local minima at $w = 2$ and $w = -1$, one local maximum at $w = 0$, and one saddle point at $w = 1$.

To identify which, if any, of these stationary points is the function's *global* minimum, we can evaluate $g(\cdot)$ at all of them and choose the one that returns the smallest output value. Here, we have that $g(2) = 1.47$, $g(1) = 1.82$, $g(0) = 2.00$,

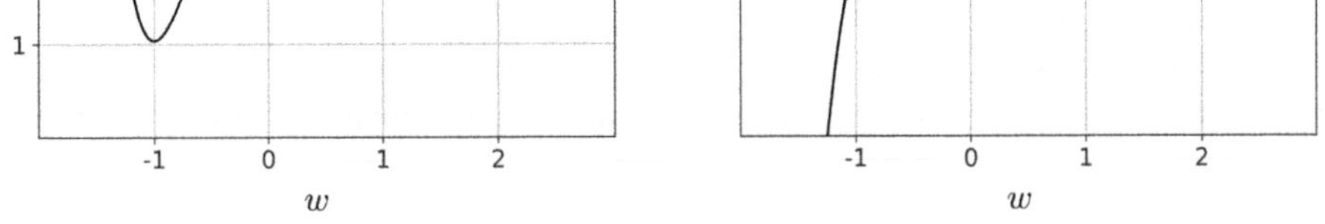

Fig. 5.5 (Left panel) The plot of the polynomial function $g(\cdot)$ defined in (5.20). (Right panel) The plot of the derivative of $g(\cdot)$ computed in (5.21). The points at which the derivative function crosses zero are its stationary points. See text for additional details

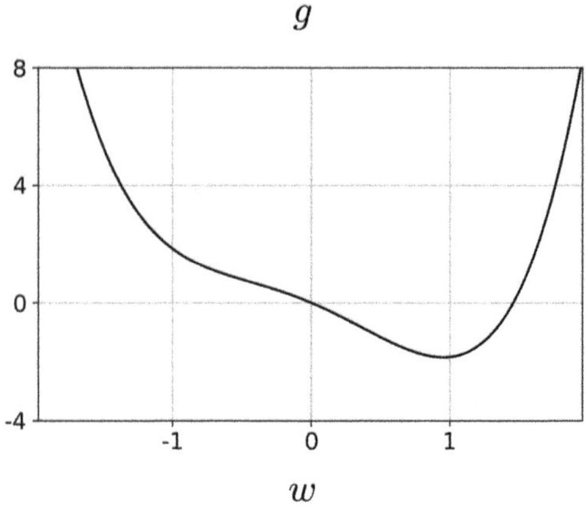

Fig. 5.6 The plot of the function $g(w) = w^4 - w^2 - w - \sin(w)$

and $g(-1) = 1.02$. In this case, $w = -1$ returns the smallest output and is therefore the function's global minimum.[4]

The fact that we were able to factorize the derivative of $g(\cdot)$ in (5.21) allowed us to determine its stationary points quickly and painlessly. This, however, is an exception rather than the rule. In general, finding a function's stationary points is not a trivial task, as we saw with the least squares and cross-entropy cost functions in (5.14) and (5.19), respectively. In such circumstances, a set of powerful numerical optimization tools can come in handy to *approximate* the stationary points. In what follows, we describe, via a simple example, one of the most commonly used numerical optimization techniques in machine learning and deep learning: the gradient descent algorithm.

Here, we introduce the gradient descent algorithm in a slow, step-by-step fashion in pursuit of minimizing the function

$$g(w) = w^4 - w^2 - w - \sin(w), \tag{5.22}$$

whose plot is shown in Fig. 5.6, and whose derivative

$$\frac{dg}{dw} = 4w^3 - 2w - 1 - \cos(w) \tag{5.23}$$

has no easy-to-identify zeros. To estimate the stationary points of $g(\cdot)$ (or equivalently the zeros of its derivative), the gradient descent algorithm is initialized at a random point $w^{[0]}$, which is then refined repeatedly through a series of mathematically defined *steps* until a reasonable approximate solution is reached.

[4] Note that this argument only works when the function $g(\cdot)$ is bounded from below. All of the cost functions introduced in this book, including but not limited to the least squares and cross-entropy cost functions we have seen so far, are specifically designed to be non-negative over their input domain and are thus bounded from below.

Here, we start the algorithm at $w^{[0]} = 0$ and use $g'(\cdot)$ to denote the derivative of $g(\cdot)$ for notational convenience. Since $g'(0) = -2$ does not happen to be zero, $w^{[0]}$ is not a minimum of $g(\cdot)$ and the algorithm will continue.

Next, we search for a new point denoted by $w^{[1]}$ that has to be a better approximation of the function's minimum than $w^{[0]}$. In other words, we aim to refine and replace $w^{[0]}$ with $w^{[1]}$ such that $g(w^{[1]}) < g(w^{[0]})$. The question then becomes whether we should move to the left or right of $w^{[0]}$ to search for $w^{[1]}$. Luckily, the answer to this question is hidden in the mathematical definition of the derivative. Recall from basic calculus that the derivative of the function $g'(\cdot)$ at $w^{[0]}$ can be approximated as

$$g'(w^{[0]}) \approx \frac{g(w^{[0]} + \varepsilon) - g(w^{[0]})}{\varepsilon}, \tag{5.24}$$

where ε is a small positive number.[5] When $g'(w^{[0]})$ is negative (as is the case here), we have that $g(w^{[0]} + \varepsilon) < g(w^{[0]})$. Hence, stepping ε units to the right of $w^{[0]}$ would decrease the evaluation of $g(\cdot)$. On the other hand, when $g'(w^{[0]})$ is positive, we should move in the opposite direction (i.e., to the left) in order to reduce the value of $g(\cdot)$. Using the mathematical sign function, we can combine these two cases together and conclude that the point

$$w^{[1]} = w^{[0]} - \varepsilon \,\text{sign}\left(g'(w^{[0]})\right) \tag{5.25}$$

approximates the minimum of $g(\cdot)$ more closely than $w^{[0]}$. Noting that $\text{sign}(t) = \frac{t}{|t|}$, we can rewrite (5.25) as

$$w^{[1]} = w^{[0]} - \alpha^{[0]} g'\left(w^{[0]}\right), \tag{5.26}$$

where we have denoted the term $\frac{\varepsilon}{|g'(w^{[0]})|}$ by $\alpha^{[0]}$ that is typically referred to as the *learning rate* in the parlance of machine learning. The elegance of the formula for updating $w^{[0]}$ in (5.26) is in the fact that it can be reused in a recursive manner to update $w^{[1]}$ itself. At $w^{[1]}$, if the derivative of $g(\cdot)$ remains negative, we continue moving to the right in pursuit of an even better approximation to the function's minimum. Otherwise, if the derivative of $g(\cdot)$ suddenly becomes positive at $w^{[1]}$, it means that we have skipped the minimum that now lies to the left of $w^{[1]}$. Again, and in either case,

$$w^{[2]} = w^{[1]} - \alpha^{[1]} g'\left(w^{[1]}\right) \tag{5.27}$$

[5] In general, the smaller the value of ε the better the approximation. In the limit, and as $\varepsilon \rightarrow 0$, we have strict equality.

Table 5.1 The sequence of points created by the gradient descent algorithm to find the minimum of the function $g(w) = w^4 - w^2 - w - \sin(w)$. The learning rate $\alpha^{[k]}$ is set to 0.1 for all iterations of the algorithm

k	$w^{[k]}$	$\alpha^{[k]}$	$g'(w^{[k]})$	$w^{[k+1]} = w^{[k]} - \alpha^{[k]}\, g'(w^{[k]})$
0	0.0000	0.1	−2.0000	0.2000
1	0.2000	0.1	−2.3481	0.4348
2	0.4348	0.1	−2.4478	0.6796
3	0.6796	0.1	−1.8816	0.8677
4	0.8677	0.1	−0.7685	0.9446
5	0.9446	0.1	−0.1040	0.9550
6	0.9550	0.1	−0.0038	0.9554
7	0.9554	0.1	-8.8×10^{-5}	0.9554
8	0.9554	0.1	-2.0×10^{-6}	0.9554
9	0.9554	0.1	-4.7×10^{-8}	0.9554

would get us closer to the true minimum of $g(\cdot)$. This process can be repeated to produce a sequence of points of the form

$$w^{[k+1]} = w^{[k]} - \alpha^{[k]}\, g'\left(w^{[k]}\right), \tag{5.28}$$

which eventually converges to the function's minimum as k grows larger. For simplicity, we can keep the learning rate $\alpha^{[k]}$ fixed at some small value (e.g., 0.1) for all k and use (5.28) to produce the sequence of points displayed in Table 5.1.

As can be seen in Table 5.1, as k increases, the derivative of the function at $w^{[k]}$ tends to shrink in magnitude, until at some point the term $\alpha^{[k]}\, g'(w^{[k]})$ becomes so close to zero that the difference between successive updates vanishes effectively, and the gradient descent algorithm converges to the point $w = 0.9554$ as the (approximate) minimum of $g(w) = w^4 - w^2 - w - \sin(w)$.

The choice of the learning rate $\alpha^{[k]}$ is important to the overall speed and performance of the gradient descent algorithm. Recall from (5.24) that the smaller the value of ε, the better the approximation. Given that ε and the learning rates are directly proportional, $\alpha^{[k]}$ should ideally be as small as possible for the gradient descent algorithm to work properly. If $\alpha^{[k]}$ is set too large, the approximation in (5.24) will no longer hold, and the gradient descent algorithm may diverge. To show how increasing the learning rate could impact the algorithm negatively, in Table 5.2 we summarize the results of applying gradient descent to minimizing $g(\cdot)$, this time using an elevated learning rate of $\alpha^{[k]} = 1.0$.

As can be seen in Table 5.2, even the moderately large learning rate value of 1.0 invalidates the underlying basis of the gradient descent in (5.24), causing the algorithm to explode within just a few iterations.

Conversely, it is also problematic if we set the learning rate too small. While very small learning rates can guarantee the gradient descent algorithm to behave properly, a very large number of iterations or steps may be needed to recover the function's

Table 5.2 The sequence of points created by the gradient descent algorithm to find the minimum of the function $g(w) = w^4 - w^2 - w - \sin(w)$. The learning rate $\alpha^{[k]}$ is set to 1.0 for all iterations of the algorithm. Here, ∞ represent numbers larger than the computational capacity of an average computer

k	$w^{[k]}$	$\alpha^{[k]}$	$g'(w^{[k]})$	$w^{[k+1]}$
0	0.0	1.0	−2.0	2.0
1	2.0	1.0	27.4	−25.4
2	−25.4	1.0	−65624.5	65599.1
3	65599.1	1.0	-1.1×10^{15}	1.1×10^{15}
4	1.1×10^{15}	1.0	-5.8×10^{45}	5.8×10^{45}
5	5.8×10^{45}	1.0	7.6×10^{137}	-7.6×10^{137}
6	-7.6×10^{137}	1.0	$-\infty$	$+\infty$

stationary point. As a general rule of thumb, the smaller the learning rate is set the lower the speed of convergence to the minimum. In Table 5.3, we summarize the results of applying gradient descent to minimizing the function $g(\cdot)$ in (5.23) using the relatively small learning rate of $\alpha^{[k]} = 0.01$. Because the learning rate is set too small in this case, we will need over 100 iterations of the algorithm to get within the same vicinity of the minimum as in Table 5.1.

Comparing the results reported in Tables 5.1, 5.2, and 5.3 indicates that choosing learning rate for gradient descent must be handled with care. Otherwise, the algorithm could either fail to converge to a minimum, or do so at a very slow pace. It must be noted that a number of advanced variants of the gradient descent algorithm exist wherein the learning rate is set automatically by the algorithm and adjusted adaptively at each iteration by leveraging the local geometry of the cost function. The inner-workings of these advanced algorithms are, for the most part, outside the scope of this book. The interested reader is encouraged to consult [8] and references therein.

Linear Classification with Multi-Dimensional Input

In this section, we extend the linear classification framework to handle general multi-dimensional input. Recall from our discussion of linear classification with one-dimensional input in Sect. "Linear Classification with One-Dimensional Input" that a linear classifier with scalar input x can be modeled as $h(f(x))$, where $h(\cdot)$ is the Heaviside step function defined in (5.2), and $f(x) = w_0 + w_1 x$ is a linear model in x, having w_0 and w_1 as tunable parameters. We then addressed the non-differentiability of $h(f(x))$ by introducing the logistic function $\sigma(\cdot)$ in (5.4), culminating in the derivation of the cross-entropy cost in (5.18). Finally, we presented the gradient descent algorithm in (5.28) as a means to minimize the cross-entropy cost and determine optimal model parameters.

Table 5.3 The sequence of points created by the gradient descent algorithm to find the minimum of the function $g(w) = w^4 - w^2 - w - \sin(w)$. The learning rate $\alpha^{[k]}$ is set to 0.01 for all iterations of the algorithm

k	$w^{[k]}$	$\alpha^{[k]}$	$g'(w^{[k]})$	$w^{[k+1]}$	k	$w^{[k]}$	$\alpha^{[k]}$	$g'(w^{[k]})$	$w^{[k+1]}$
0	0	0.01	−2.0000	0.0200	50	0.9063	0.01	−0.4515	0.9108
1	0.0200	0.01	−2.0398	0.0404	51	0.9108	0.01	−0.4123	0.9149
2	0.0404	0.01	−2.0797	0.0612	52	0.9149	0.01	−0.3760	0.9187
3	0.0612	0.01	−2.1196	0.0824	53	0.9187	0.01	−0.3426	0.9221
4	0.0824	0.01	−2.1592	0.1040	54	0.9221	0.01	−0.3119	0.9253
5	0.1040	0.01	−2.1981	0.1260	55	0.9253	0.01	−0.2837	0.9281
6	0.1260	0.01	−2.2360	0.1483	56	0.9281	0.01	−0.2579	0.9307
7	0.1483	0.01	−2.2726	0.1710	57	0.9307	0.01	−0.2343	0.9330
8	0.1710	0.01	−2.3075	0.1941	58	0.9330	0.01	−0.2127	0.9351
9	0.1941	0.01	−2.3402	0.2175	59	0.9351	0.01	−0.1929	0.9371
10	0.2175	0.01	−2.3703	0.2412	60	0.9371	0.01	−0.1750	0.9388
11	0.2412	0.01	−2.3974	0.2652	61	0.9388	0.01	−0.1586	0.9404
12	0.2652	0.01	−2.4208	0.2894	62	0.9404	0.01	−0.1437	0.9418
13	0.2894	0.01	−2.4403	0.3138	63	0.9418	0.01	−0.1301	0.9431
14	0.3138	0.01	−2.4552	0.3384	64	0.9431	0.01	−0.1178	0.9443
15	0.3384	0.01	−2.4651	0.3630	65	0.9443	0.01	−0.1066	0.9454
16	0.3630	0.01	−2.4695	0.3877	66	0.9454	0.01	−0.0964	0.9463
17	0.3877	0.01	−2.4681	0.4124	67	0.9463	0.01	−0.0872	0.9472
18	0.4124	0.01	−2.4604	0.4370	68	0.9472	0.01	−0.0789	0.9480
19	0.4370	0.01	−2.4462	0.4615	69	0.9480	0.01	−0.0713	0.9487
20	0.4615	0.01	−2.4253	0.4857	70	0.9487	0.01	−0.0645	0.9494
21	0.4857	0.01	−2.3974	0.5097	71	0.9494	0.01	−0.0583	0.9500
22	0.5097	0.01	−2.3626	0.5333	72	0.9500	0.01	−0.0527	0.9505
23	0.5333	0.01	−2.3210	0.5565	73	0.9505	0.01	−0.0476	0.9510
24	0.5565	0.01	−2.2727	0.5792	74	0.9510	0.01	−0.0430	0.9514
25	0.5792	0.01	−2.2180	0.6014	75	0.9514	0.01	−0.0388	0.9518
26	0.6014	0.01	−2.1572	0.6230	76	0.9518	0.01	−0.0351	0.9521
27	0.6230	0.01	−2.0909	0.6439	77	0.9521	0.01	−0.0317	0.9524
28	0.6439	0.01	−2.0197	0.6641	78	0.9524	0.01	−0.0286	0.9527
29	0.6641	0.01	−1.9441	0.6835	79	0.9527	0.01	−0.0258	0.9530
30	0.6835	0.01	−1.8649	0.7022	80	0.9530	0.01	−0.0233	0.9532
31	0.7022	0.01	−1.7829	0.7200	81	0.9532	0.01	−0.0211	0.9534
32	0.7200	0.01	−1.6987	0.7370	82	0.9534	0.01	−0.0190	0.9536
33	0.7370	0.01	−1.6132	0.7531	83	0.9536	0.01	−0.0172	0.9538
34	0.7531	0.01	−1.5270	0.7684	84	0.9538	0.01	−0.0155	0.9539
35	0.7684	0.01	−1.4410	0.7828	85	0.9539	0.01	−0.0140	0.9541
36	0.7828	0.01	−1.3557	0.7964	86	0.9541	0.01	−0.0126	0.9542
37	0.7964	0.01	−1.2717	0.8091	87	0.9542	0.01	−0.0114	0.9543
38	0.8091	0.01	−1.1897	0.8210	88	0.9543	0.01	−0.0103	0.9544
39	0.8210	0.01	−1.1100	0.8321	89	0.9544	0.01	−0.0093	0.9545
40	0.8321	0.01	−1.0330	0.8424	90	0.9545	0.01	−0.0084	0.9546

(continued)

Table 5.3 (continued)

k	$w^{[k]}$	$\alpha^{[k]}$	$g'(w^{[k]})$	$w^{[k+1]}$	k	$w^{[k]}$	$\alpha^{[k]}$	$g'(w^{[k]})$	$w^{[k+1]}$
41	0.8424	0.01	−0.9591	0.8520	91	0.9546	0.01	−0.0076	0.9547
42	0.8520	0.01	−0.8885	0.8609	92	0.9547	0.01	−0.0068	0.9547
43	0.8609	0.01	−0.8213	0.8691	93	0.9547	0.01	−0.0062	0.9548
44	0.8691	0.01	−0.7578	0.8767	94	0.9548	0.01	−0.0056	0.9549
45	0.8767	0.01	−0.6978	0.8837	95	0.9549	0.01	−0.0050	0.9549
46	0.8837	0.01	−0.6415	0.8901	96	0.9549	0.01	−0.0045	0.9550
47	0.8901	0.01	−0.5888	0.8960	97	0.9550	0.01	−0.0041	0.9550
48	0.8960	0.01	−0.5397	0.9014	98	0.9550	0.01	−0.0037	0.9550
49	0.9014	0.01	−0.4939	0.9063	99	0.9550	0.01	−0.0033	0.9551

Each of the steps described above can be adjusted slightly to accommodate an n-dimensional input vector $\mathbf{x}$. First, as we saw previously in Sect. "Linear Regression with Multi-Dimensional Input", the linear function $f(\cdot)$ with $\mathbf{x}$ as input can be written as

$$f(\mathbf{x}) = w_0 + \mathbf{w}^T\,\mathbf{x} \tag{5.29}$$

with the scalar w_0 and the $n \times 1$ vector $\mathbf{w}$ as parameters. It is notationally convenient to temporarily redefine the vectors $\mathbf{x}$ and $\mathbf{w}$ to include 1 and w_0 as their first entry, respectively, and write (5.29) even more compactly as

$$f(\mathbf{x}) = \mathbf{w}^T\,\mathbf{x}. \tag{5.30}$$

Next, the cross-entropy cost can be derived similarly as

$$g(\mathbf{w}) = -\frac{1}{p}\sum_{i=1}^{p} y_i \log\left(\sigma(\mathbf{w}^T\mathbf{x}_i)\right) + (1-y_i)\log\left(1-\sigma(\mathbf{w}^T\mathbf{x}_i)\right). \tag{5.31}$$

As its name suggests, gradient descent is a *gradient*-based algorithm. When dealing with vectors, the gradient descent update formula in (5.28) can be modified as

$$\mathbf{w}^{[k+1]} = \mathbf{w}^{[k]} - \alpha^{[k]}\,\nabla g\left(\mathbf{w}^{[k]}\right), \tag{5.32}$$

where the scalar $w^{[k]}$ is replaced by its vector analog $\mathbf{w}^{[k]}$, and the derivative function $g'(\cdot)$ is replaced by the gradient function $\nabla g(\cdot)$. As discussed previously, the gradient descent algorithm can be initialized at any random point $\mathbf{w}^{[0]}$, and refined sequentially using (5.32) until a "good enough" approximation of the function's minimum is reached. In practice, we halt the algorithm after a maximum number of iterations are taken or when the norm of the gradient has fallen below some small user-defined value, whichever comes first (Fig. 5.7).

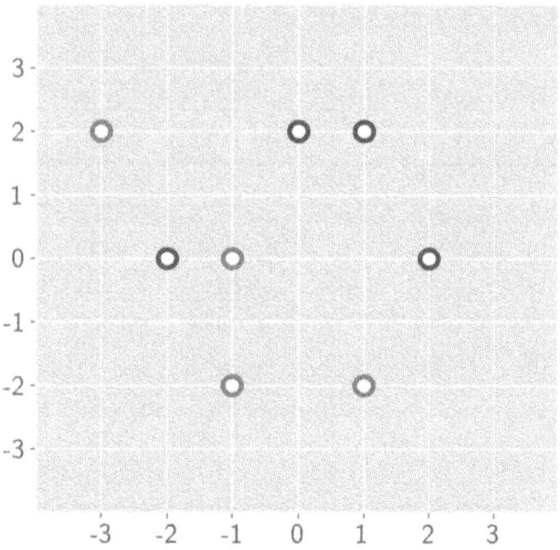

Fig. 5.7 The input-space illustration of the classification dataset in (5.33). Here, each input point is color-coded based on its output value, where the color red is used to indicate the points belonging to class "0" and blue is used to indicate the points belonging to class "1"

Example 5.1 (Linear Classification of a Simulated Dataset) In this example, we train a linear classifier for a simulated dataset consisting of $p = 8$ data points of the form $(\mathbf{x}_i, y_i)$

$$\left(\begin{bmatrix}1\\-2\end{bmatrix},0\right),\ \left(\begin{bmatrix}-1\\0\end{bmatrix},0\right),\ \left(\begin{bmatrix}-3\\2\end{bmatrix},0\right),\ \left(\begin{bmatrix}-1\\-2\end{bmatrix},0\right),$$
$$\left(\begin{bmatrix}1\\2\end{bmatrix},1\right),\ \left(\begin{bmatrix}0\\2\end{bmatrix},1\right),\ \left(\begin{bmatrix}2\\0\end{bmatrix},1\right),\ \left(\begin{bmatrix}-2\\0\end{bmatrix},1\right), \tag{5.33}$$

where $\mathbf{x}_i$ is a two-dimensional input and y_i is a binary output. This particular dataset is plotted in Fig. 5.9.

To use the gradient descent algorithm, we must first find the functional form of the gradient of the cross-entropy cost function in (5.31), which as you will show in Exercise 5.5 is given by

$$\nabla g(\mathbf{w}) = \frac{1}{p}\sum_{i=1}^{p}\left(\sigma(\mathbf{w}^T\mathbf{x}_i) - y_i\right)\mathbf{x}_i. \tag{5.34}$$

To choose a proper learning rate for gradient descent, it is advisable to run the algorithm for a limited number of iterations using a range of different values for $\alpha^{[k]}$ and plot the resulting cost function evaluations at each step. We have done so in the left panel of Fig. 5.8 for three learning rate values: 10, 1, and 0.1. As can be seen in the figure, $\alpha^{[k]} = 10$ is evidently too large, causing the algorithm to diverge. The learning rate of 0.1 is too small on the other hand,

(continued)

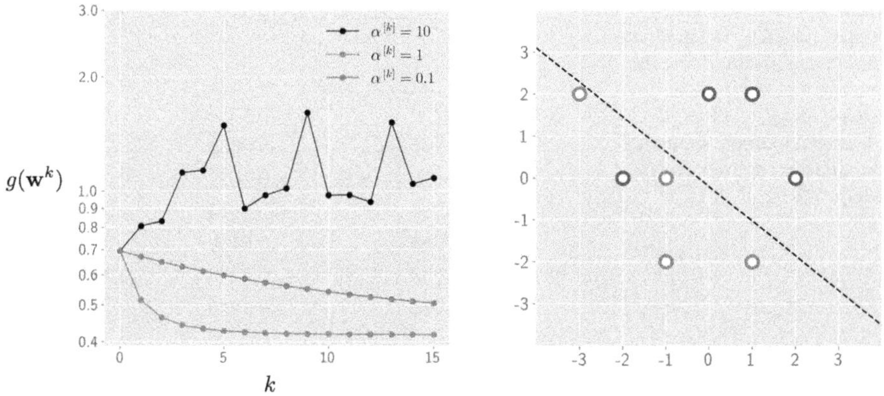

Fig. 5.8 (Left panel) The cost function evaluations resulted from three runs of gradient descent for minimizing the cross-entropy cost associated with the dataset in Fig. 5.9. The runs were initiated at the same starting point, but with different learning rates. The vertical axis is logarithmic in scale. (Right panel) The linear boundary separating the two classes of data is characterized by the equation in (5.36) and drawn as a dashed black line

Example 5.1 (continued)
as it causes the evaluation of the cost function to decline ever so slowly. In contrast, a learning rate of 1 seems to be ideal for the dataset at hand.

Initializing gradient descent at $\mathbf{w}^{[0]} = \mathbf{0}_{3\times 1}$ with $\alpha^{[k]} = 1$, we run the algorithm in (5.32) for a total of 100 iterations, storing the results along the way in Table 5.4. Note that the norm of the gradient falls below 10^{-5} near the bottom of the table, indicating that the last recorded point, i.e.,

$$\mathbf{w}^{[99]} = \begin{bmatrix} 0.2184 \\ 0.9107 \\ 1.1016 \end{bmatrix}, \tag{5.35}$$

is in close proximity of the true minimum of the cost function. The classification boundary can then be written as

$$f(x_1, x_2) = 0.2184 + 0.9107\,x_1 + 1.1016\,x_2 = 0 \tag{5.36}$$

and plotted as illustrated in the right panel of Fig. 5.8.

Table 5.4 The sequence of points created by the gradient descent algorithm to find the minimum of the cross-entropy cost function associated with the simulated classification dataset shown in Fig. 5.9

k	$\mathbf{w}^{[k]}$	$\alpha^{[k]}$	$\nabla g(\mathbf{w}^{[k]})$	$\|\nabla g(\mathbf{w}^{[k]})\|$
0	$\begin{bmatrix} 0 \\ 0 \\ 0 \end{bmatrix}$	1.0	$\begin{bmatrix} 0 \\ -0.3125 \\ -0.3750 \end{bmatrix}$	0.4881
1	$\begin{bmatrix} 0 \\ 0.3125 \\ 0.3750 \end{bmatrix}$	1.0	$\begin{bmatrix} -0.0066 \\ -0.1623 \\ -0.1934 \end{bmatrix}$	0.2525
2	$\begin{bmatrix} 0.0066 \\ 0.4748 \\ 0.5684 \end{bmatrix}$	1.0	$\begin{bmatrix} -0.0100 \\ -0.0978 \\ -0.1215 \end{bmatrix}$	0.1563
$\vdots$	$\vdots$	$\vdots$	$\vdots$	$\vdots$
98	$\begin{bmatrix} 0.2184 \\ 0.9107 \\ 1.1016 \end{bmatrix}$	1.0	$\begin{bmatrix} -3.4 \times 10^{-6} \\ -1.7 \times 10^{-6} \\ -1.3 \times 10^{-6} \end{bmatrix}$	4.0×10^{-6}
99	$\begin{bmatrix} 0.2184 \\ 0.9107 \\ 1.1016 \end{bmatrix}$	1.0	$\begin{bmatrix} -3.1 \times 10^{-6} \\ -1.6 \times 10^{-6} \\ -1.2 \times 10^{-6} \end{bmatrix}$	3.7×10^{-6}

Linear Classification with Multiple Classes

So far in the chapter, we have focused our attention on *binary* classification where the output takes on only one of two possible values or outcomes. In practice, however, classification problems with more than two classes are just as common as their binary counterparts. For instance, in many oncology applications, we are interested in classifying certain tissue images into one of three categories: "normal," "benign," or "malignant." Once a cancer diagnosis is made, we may be interested in evaluating its aggressiveness by assigning it one of *four* pathological grades: "low-grade" (G1), "intermediate-grade" (G2), "high-grade" (G3), or "anaplastic" (G4). The higher the tumor grade the more quickly it grows and spreads throughout the body. Hence, accurate tumor grading is key to devising the optimal treatment approach.

In this section, we discuss how the binary classification framework we developed previously can be extended to handle multi-class problems such as the examples mentioned above. In general, a multi-class classification problem involves $m > 2$ classes. Focusing on the jth class for the moment, we already know how to differentiate it from the *rest of the data* using a binary classifier. This can be done by lumping together every other class of data (except the jth one) into a new category called the "not j" class. Next, we temporarily assign the label "1" to the jth class and the label "0" to the "not j" class and train a linear classifier to separate the two as discussed in Example 5.1. Denoting the bias and slope parameters of this linear classifier by $w_{0,j}$ and $\mathbf{w}_j$, the equation of the separating boundary can be written as

$$f_j(\mathbf{x}) = w_{0,j} + \mathbf{w}_j^T \mathbf{x} = 0. \tag{5.37}$$

It can be shown, using elementary linear algebra calculations, that the expression

$$\mathcal{D}_j(\mathbf{x}) = \frac{f_j(\mathbf{x})}{\|\mathbf{w}_j\|} = \frac{w_{0,j} + \mathbf{w}_j^T \mathbf{x}}{\|\mathbf{w}_j\|} \tag{5.38}$$

computes the distance from the input point $\mathbf{x}$ to the linear boundary in (5.37). The distance metric in (5.38) is positive if $\mathbf{x}$ lies on the positive side of the boundary (where class "1" resides) and negative when $\mathbf{x}$ falls on the negative side of the boundary (where class "0" resides).

Repeating the process outlined above m times, once for each class of data, we end up with the m linear functions $f_1(\cdot)$ through $f_m(\cdot)$. We can then use these functions to compute the m corresponding distance values $\mathcal{D}_1$ through $\mathcal{D}_m$. The index associated with the largest distance

$$y = \underset{j=1,\ldots,m}{\operatorname{argmax}} \; \mathcal{D}_j(\mathbf{x}) \tag{5.39}$$

determines the output of $\mathbf{x}$. The expression in (5.39) is sometimes referred to as the *one-versus-rest* classifier.

Example 5.2 (Linear Classification of a Multi-class Dataset) In this example, we train a multi-class classifier for the following simulated dataset consisting of $p = 12$ data points of the form $(\mathbf{x}_i, y_i)$

$$\begin{aligned}
&\left(\begin{bmatrix}-2\\1\end{bmatrix}, 1\right), \left(\begin{bmatrix}-3\\1\end{bmatrix}, 1\right), \left(\begin{bmatrix}-3\\-2\end{bmatrix}, 1\right), \left(\begin{bmatrix}-2\\0\end{bmatrix}, 1\right),\\
&\left(\begin{bmatrix}1\\-1\end{bmatrix}, 2\right), \left(\begin{bmatrix}2\\-2\end{bmatrix}, 2\right), \left(\begin{bmatrix}3\\0\end{bmatrix}, 2\right), \left(\begin{bmatrix}0\\-3\end{bmatrix}, 2\right),\\
&\left(\begin{bmatrix}2\\2\end{bmatrix}, 3\right), \left(\begin{bmatrix}1\\2\end{bmatrix}, 3\right), \left(\begin{bmatrix}1\\3\end{bmatrix}, 3\right), \left(\begin{bmatrix}2\\3\end{bmatrix}, 3\right),
\end{aligned} \tag{5.40}$$

where the input $\mathbf{x}_i$ is two-dimensional, and the output y_i is equal to either 1, 2, or 3. This particular dataset is plotted in Fig. 5.9.

First, we train a linear classifier to separate class "1" from the rest of the data. Following the process set forth in Example 5.1, the linear boundary associated with this binary classification subproblem can be defined as $f_1(\mathbf{x}) = w_{0,1} + \mathbf{w}_1^T \mathbf{x} = 0$, with the parameters $w_{0,1}$ and $\mathbf{w}_1$ recovered using gradient descent as

(continued)

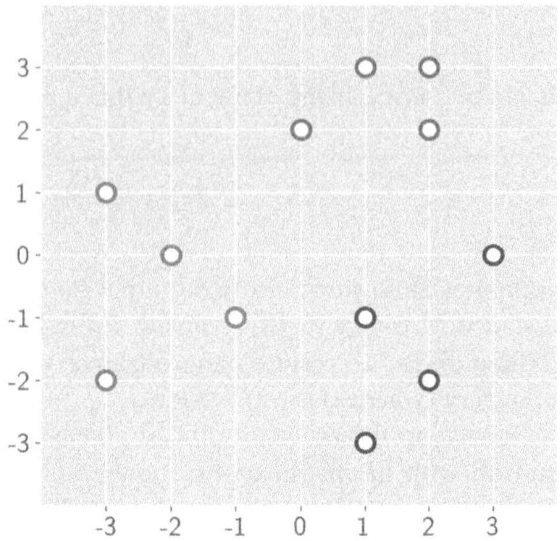

Fig. 5.9 The input-space illustration of the classification dataset in (5.40). Here, each input point is color-coded based on its output value, with the colors red, blue, and green highlighting the points belonging to the classes "1," "2," and "3," respectively

Example 5.2 (continued)

$$w_{0,1} = -3.56, \qquad \mathbf{w}_1 = \begin{bmatrix} -5.82 \\ 0.88 \end{bmatrix}. \tag{5.41}$$

The parameters of $f_2(\cdot)$ and $f_3(\cdot)$ can be found similarly as

$$\begin{aligned} w_{0,2} &= -3.87, & \mathbf{w}_2 &= \begin{bmatrix} 4.46 \\ -5.45 \end{bmatrix}, \\ w_{0,3} &= -8.19, & \mathbf{w}_3 &= \begin{bmatrix} 1.10 \\ 6.29 \end{bmatrix}. \end{aligned} \tag{5.42}$$

Finally, the distance function associated with each binary classifier can be computed via (5.38) as

$$\begin{aligned} \mathcal{D}_1 &= -0.60 - 0.99\,x_1 + 0.15\,x_2, \\ \mathcal{D}_2 &= -0.55 + 0.63\,x_1 - 0.77\,x_2, \\ \mathcal{D}_3 &= -1.28 + 0.17\,x_1 + 0.99\,x_2. \end{aligned} \tag{5.43}$$

Figure 5.10 shows the multi-class classification boundaries characterized by the rule in (5.39) and the distance functions derived in (5.43).

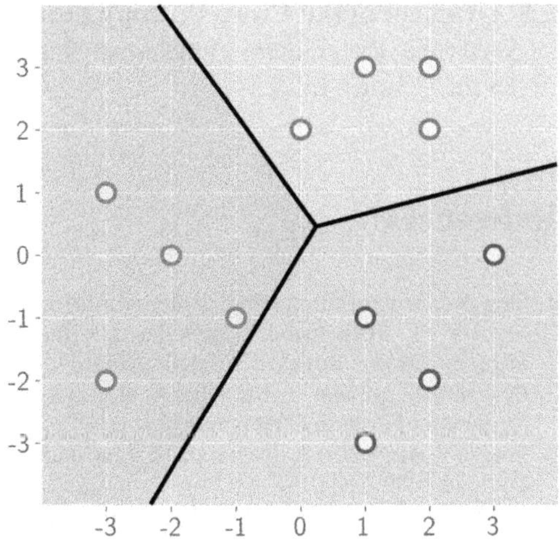

Fig. 5.10 The input-space illustration of the classification dataset in (5.40) along with the separating boundaries defined by the distance functions in (5.43). Notice, in particular, that the three black line segments converge at the point (0.24, 0.48) where $\mathcal{D}_1 = \mathcal{D}_2 = \mathcal{D}_3$

Problems

5.1 Solving a Classification Problem Using Linear Regression

Follow the steps outlined in Example 4.1 to find the best linear regression fit for the classification data in (5.1).

5.2 Stationary Points of the Cross-Entropy Cost Function

Verify that setting the partial derivatives of the cross-entropy cost function in (5.18) yields the system of equations shown in (5.19).

5.3 The Logistic Function

(a) Use the definition of the logistic function $\sigma(\cdot)$ in (5.4) to show that the properties expressed in (5.7), (5.8), and (5.10) indeed hold.
(b) For what value of K does the logistic sigmoid function become a solution to the differential equation in (5.6)?
(c) In general, how would you adjust the definition of $\sigma(t)$ so that it is always a solution to (5.6) regardless of the value of K?

5.4 Gradient Descent

Apply the gradient descent algorithm to find the minimum of the polynomial function

$$g(w) = w^6 - w^5 + w^4 - w \tag{5.44}$$

using a learning rate value of

(a) $\alpha = 10$.
(b) $\alpha = 0.1$.
(c) $\alpha = 0.01$.

5.5 Gradient of the Cross-Entropy Function
Verify that the gradient of the cross-entropy cost function in (5.31) can be written in the form shown in (5.34).

References

1. Shor NZ. Minimization methods for non-differentiable functions. Berlin: Springer; 1985
2. Verhulst PF. Mathematical researches into the law of population growth increase. Nouveaux Mires de l'Acade Royale des Sciences et Belles-Lettres de Bruxelles. 1845;18:8
3. Benzekry S, Lamont C, Beheshti A, et al. Classical mathematical models for description and prediction of experimental tumor growth. PLoS Comput Biol. 2014;10(8):e100380
4. Vaidya V, Alexandro F. Evaluation of some mathematical models for tumor growth. Int J Biomed Comput. 1982;13(1):19–36
5. Hsieh Y, Lee J, Chang H. SARS epidemiology modeling. Emerg Infect Dis. 2004;10(6):11651168
6. Wang P, Zheng X, Li J, et al. Prediction of epidemic trends in COVID-19 with logistic model and machine learning techniques. Chaos, Solitons Fractals. 2020;139:110058
7. The World Health Organization (WHO) COVID-19 global dataset. Accessed Apr 2022. https://covid19.who.int/data
8. Watt J, Borhani R, Katsaggelos AK. Machine learning refined: foundations, algorithms, and applications. Cambridge: Cambridge University Press; 2020

Chapter 6
From Feature Engineering to Deep Learning

The models we have studied thus far in the book have all been linear. In this chapter, we begin our foray into nonlinear models by formally introducing features as mathematical functions that transform the input data. We discuss two main approaches to defining features: *feature engineering* that is driven by the domain knowledge of human experts and *feature learning* that is fully driven by the data itself. A discussion of the latter approach naturally leads to the introduction of deep neural networks as the main driver of recent advances in the field.

Feature Engineering for Nonlinear Regression

In Sect. "Linear Regression with Multi-Dimensional Input", we studied the linear model for regression that takes the form

$$f(x_1, x_2, \ldots, x_n) = w_0 + w_1x_1 + w_2x_2 + \cdots + w_nx_n, \tag{6.1}$$

or, more compactly,

$$f(\mathbf{x}) = w_0 + \mathbf{w}^T\mathbf{x} \tag{6.2}$$

if we arrange all the inputs x_1 through x_n into a single input vector denoted as

$$\mathbf{x} = \begin{bmatrix} x_1 \\ x_2 \\ \vdots \\ x_n \end{bmatrix}, \tag{6.3}$$

and all the parameters w_1 through w_n into a single parameter vector denoted as

R. Borhani et al., *Fundamentals of Machine Learning and Deep Learning in Medicine*, https://doi.org/10.1007/978-3-031-19502-0_6

$$\mathbf{w} = \begin{bmatrix} w_1 \\ w_2 \\ \vdots \\ w_n \end{bmatrix}. \tag{6.4}$$

For many real-world regression datasets, however, the linear model in (6.2) is not capable of capturing the complex *nonlinear* relationship that may exist between the input and the output. One way to solve this issue is by injecting nonlinearity into this model via what are called *features* in the parlance of machine learning. A feature $h(\mathbf{x})$ is a nonlinear mathematical function of the input $\mathbf{x}$. For instance,

$$h(x_1, x_2, \ldots, x_n) = x_1^2 + x_2^2 + \cdots + x_n^2 \tag{6.5}$$

is a polynomial feature of the input, whereas

$$h(x_1, x_2, \ldots, x_n) = \cos(x_1) \tag{6.6}$$

is a trigonometric one. Notice from (6.6) that a feature does not necessarily have to involve all the inputs x_1 through x_n, but in general it can. A nonlinear regression model, in general, can employ m such features h_1 through h_m

$$f(\mathbf{x}) = v_0 + v_1 h_1(\mathbf{x}) + v_2 h_2(\mathbf{x}) + \cdots + v_m h_m(\mathbf{x}), \tag{6.7}$$

which can be written more compactly as

$$f(\mathbf{x}) = v_0 + \mathbf{v}^T \mathbf{h}(\mathbf{x}) \tag{6.8}$$

denoting

$$\mathbf{v} = \begin{bmatrix} v_1 \\ v_2 \\ \vdots \\ v_m \end{bmatrix} \tag{6.9}$$

and

$$\mathbf{h}(\mathbf{x}) = \begin{bmatrix} h_1(\mathbf{x}) \\ h_2(\mathbf{x}) \\ \vdots \\ h_m(\mathbf{x}) \end{bmatrix}. \tag{6.10}$$

Regardless of how the features in (6.10) are chosen, the steps we take to formally resolve the nonlinear regression model in (6.7) are entirely similar to what we saw in Sect. "Linear Regression with Multi-Dimensional Input" for linear regression. To briefly recap the process, we first form a least squares cost function

$$g\left(v_0, \mathbf{v}\right) = \frac{1}{p}\sum_{i=1}^{p}\left(v_0 + \mathbf{v}^T\mathbf{h}(\mathbf{x}_i) - y_i\right)^2 \tag{6.11}$$

over a regression dataset consisting of p input–output pairs $\left\{(\mathbf{x}_1, y_1), \ldots, \left(\mathbf{x}_p, y_p\right)\right\}$. We then minimize this cost function by setting the derivative of g with respect to v and the gradient of g with respect to $\mathbf{v}$ equal to zero simultaneously. Solving the resulting linear system will reveal the optimal values for v and $\mathbf{v}$. The only issue that remains is determining appropriate nonlinear functions to form the feature vector in (6.10). Let us explore this issue further through an example.

Example 6.1 (Feature Engineering for Bacterial Growth) Lactobacillus delbrueckii is a lactic acid bacterium that can cause urinary tract infections in women. Notwithstanding, this microorganism has found industrial applications as a starter in wine and yogurt production. Table 6.1 summarizes the data associated with the growth of this bacteria in spatially constrained laboratory conditions. The input of this regression dataset is the *time* measured in hours (first column), and the output is the organism's *concentration* or (mass per unit volume) measured in grams per liter (second column).

In Sect. "The Logistic Function", we discussed various models of population growth, focusing on Verhulst's logistic model of growth. This culminated in the introduction of the sigmoid function

$$\sigma(x) = \frac{1}{1 + e^{-x}}, \tag{6.12}$$

(continued)

Table 6.1 Data for *Lactobacillus delbrueckii* growth taken from [1]

Time [h]	Concentration [g/L]
0	0.229
3	0.286
6	0.503
9	1.035
12	2.070
15	2.770
18	3.320
21	3.650
24	3.610

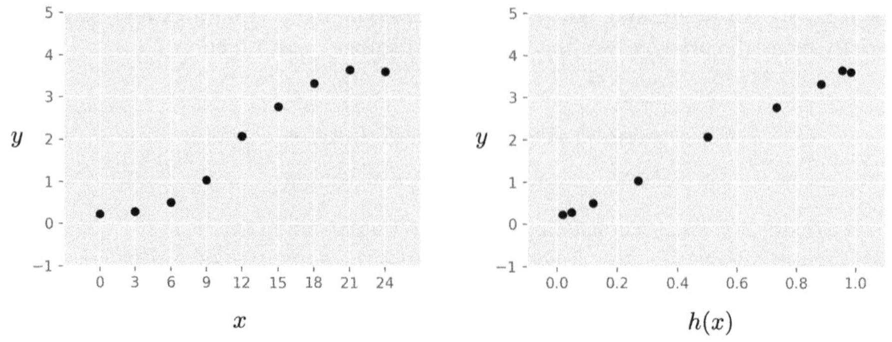

Fig. 6.1 Figure associated with Example 6.1. See text for details

Example 6.1 (continued)
which can model bacterial growth in spatially constrained environments. Using this piece of prior knowledge, we can hypothesize that transforming the input using the sigmoid function as a nonlinear feature might "linearize" this regression dataset. Figure 6.1 shows that this is indeed the case. In the left panel of the figure, we plot the original dataset provided in Table 6.1, with time along the horizontal axis and bacterial concentration along the vertical axis. In the right panel, we plot the same data, this time with the input having undergone the following nonlinear feature transformation:

$$h(x) = \sigma\left(\frac{x - 12}{3}\right). \tag{6.13}$$

Our proposed feature did its job: the input–output relationship that was nonlinear in the original space has become linear in the feature space.

In Example 6.1, we relied on what we knew about the nature of bacterial growth to determine an appropriate nonlinear feature transformation (the sigmoid function) that could linearize the relationship between the transformed input and the output. This is an instance of what is more broadly referred to as *feature engineering*, wherein the functional form of nonlinearities is determined (or engineered) by humans through their expertise, domain knowledge, intuition about the problem at hand, etc. A properly engineered feature (or a set of features) is the one that provides a good linear fit in the feature space, wherein the input has undergone nonlinear feature transformation.

Feature Engineering for Nonlinear Classification

Mirroring our treatment of feature engineering for nonlinear regression in the previous section, here we introduce the general framework of feature engineering for nonlinear classification.[1] As we saw in Sect. "Linear Classification with Multiple Classes", a linear classification boundary can be expressed algebraically as

$$f(\mathbf{x}) = w_0 + \mathbf{w}^T \mathbf{x} = 0, \tag{6.14}$$

where we have used the notation in (6.3) and (6.4) to write the equation of the boundary more compactly. When the two classes of data are not linearly separable, we can adjust this equation by injecting nonlinearity into it in an entirely similar fashion as we did in the previous section. Specifically, we replace the linear model in (6.14) with a nonlinear model of the form

$$f(\mathbf{x}) = v_0 + \mathbf{v}^T \mathbf{h}(\mathbf{x}) = 0, \tag{6.15}$$

where the weight vector $\mathbf{v}$ and the feature vector $\mathbf{h}(\mathbf{x})$ are defined in (6.9) and (6.10), respectively. Next, we need to define a proper cost function to minimize in order to resolve this nonlinear model. As discussed in Sect. "Linear Classification with Multiple Classes", one appropriate cost function to use for classification is the cross-entropy cost function that can be written in this case as

$$g(v_0, \mathbf{v}) = -\frac{1}{p} \sum_{i=1}^{p} y_i \log\left(\sigma\left(v_0 + \mathbf{v}^T \mathbf{h}\left(\mathbf{x}_i\right)\right)\right) + (1 - y_i) \log\left(1 - \sigma\left(\mathbf{w}^T \mathbf{h}\left(\mathbf{x}_i\right)\right)\right) \tag{6.16}$$

and minimized using gradient descent.

Example 6.2 (Feature Engineering for Classification) In Fig. 6.2, we show a toy classification dataset consisting of $p = 100$ two-dimensional inputs belonging to one of two classes: red or blue. It is clear from the figure that a linear model would fail to separate the two classes of data.

Here, because the input is low-dimensional, we can visually examine the data and leverage our mathematical intuition to engineer appropriate nonlinear features. In this case, the blue class seems to fall inside a circular region centered at the origin. Knowing from elementary geometry that such a circle could be represented mathematically as $x_1^2 + x_2^2 = r^2$ for some radius r, we

(continued)

[1] In this section, we only consider the case of two-class or binary classification. Multi-class classification follows similarly and is left out here to avoid repetition.

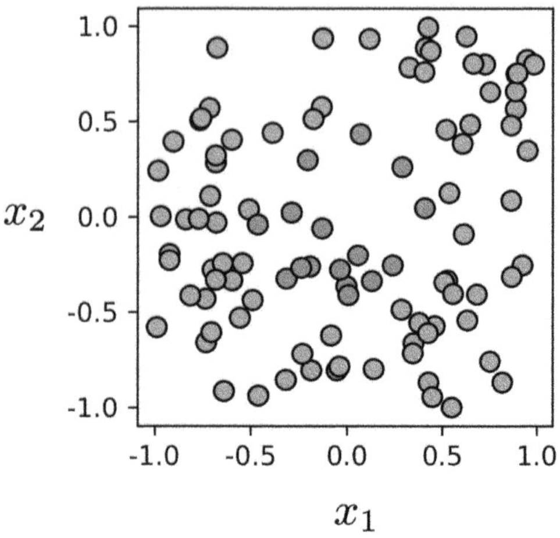

Fig. 6.2 A toy classification dataset that is not linearly separable

Example 6.2 (continued)
can propose the following nonlinear features:

$$h_1(x_1, x_2) = x_1^2,$$
$$h_2(x_1, x_2) = x_2^2. \tag{6.17}$$

As shown in Fig. 6.3, once we transform the inputs using the features defined in (6.17), the two classes of data that were not linearly separable in the original input space become linearly separable in the feature space.

Feature Learning

In Sects. "Feature Engineering for Nonlinear Regression" and "Feature Engineering for Nonlinear Classification", we described the general notion of feature engineering as a way to convert nonlinear regression and classification into linear problems. In Example 6.1, we used our mathematical knowledge of population growth in constrained environments to engineer a logistic feature that linearized the regression dataset shown in Fig. 6.1. In Example 6.2, we used our ability to visualize low-dimensional datasets to construct the quadratic features in (6.17) that helped us linearize the boundary separating the two classes of data in Fig. 6.3.

While we were successful in engineering proper features in the two examples above, in the vast majority of real-world machine learning problems, we cannot rely on these feature engineering strategies. Virtually, all modern problems of interest

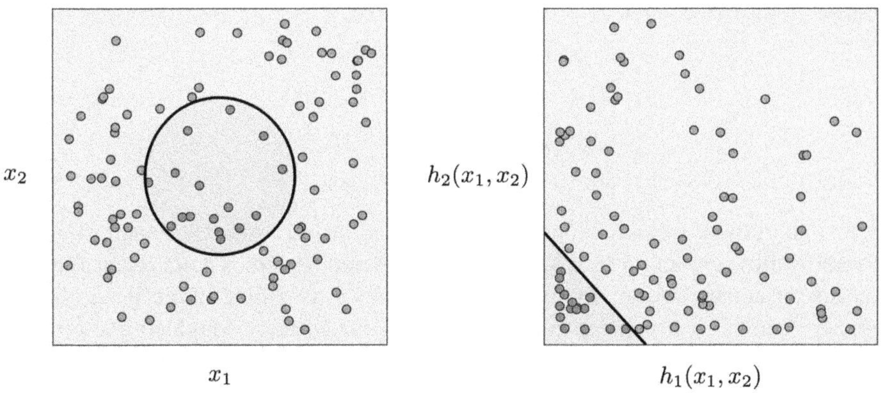

Fig. 6.3 Figure associated with Example 6.2. A well-engineered set of features as defined in (6.17) provide good nonlinear separation in the problem's original input space (left panel) and, simultaneously, good linear separation in the feature space (right panel). See text for further details

in medicine are too high-dimensional to visualize. Besides, more often than not we have too little or no knowledge of the phenomenon that governs the problem of interest. Even with prior knowledge of the phenomenon under study, the process of engineering features is non-trivial and time-consuming as it will typically involve multiple rounds of discussion and refinement between medical experts and machine learning developers [2]. Motivated by these challenges, in this section, we introduce an alternative approach to feature engineering, in which features are *learned* directly from the data itself without the need for human involvement. This new approach, commonly referred to as *feature learning*, allows us to automate the manual (and somewhat tedious) task of feature engineering.

The key idea behind feature learning is to use parameterized features in (6.7) whose parameters are tuned alongside other model parameters during training. In other words, in a feature learning setup, the nonlinear regression model in (6.7) can be adjusted and written as

$$f(\mathbf{x}) = v_0 + v_1 h_1(\mathbf{x}; \theta_1) + v_2 h_2(\mathbf{x}; \theta_2) + \cdots + v_m h_m(\mathbf{x}; \theta_m), \tag{6.18}$$

wherein θ_i represents the set of feature parameters internal to h_i. The features h_1 through h_m usually come from the same catalog or a family of functions. The most popular feature learning family of functions is the so-called *artificial neural networks* that originated in the mid-twentieth century as a rough mathematical approximation of biological neural networks. In Fig. 6.4, we show a graphical representation of an artificial neuron, which is essentially a "multi-input parameterized nonlinear" function. Let us parse the last phrase in quotations.

As illustrated in Fig. 6.4, an artificial neuron is a *multi-input* function receiving in general n inputs x_1 through x_n. It is also a *parameterized* function since each of its inputs (x_1 through x_n) is multiplied by a corresponding parameter (w_1 through w_n)

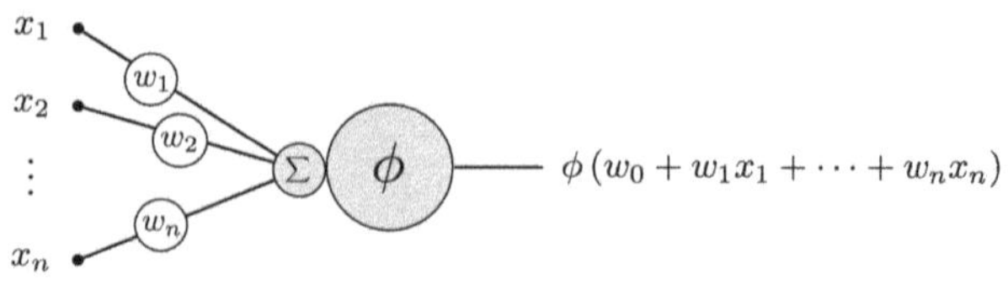

Fig. 6.4 An artificial neuron illustrated

before all of these weighted inputs are aggregated inside a summation unit shown as a small yellow circle in Fig. 6.4. Finally, an artificial neuron is a *nonlinear* function because it consists of an "activation" unit (shown as a blue circle in the figure) whose output is a nonlinear transformation of the linearly weighted combination $w_1x_1 + \cdots + w_nx_n$.[2] Stitching all the pieces together, an artificial neuron can be modeled as

$$h(x_1, x_2, \ldots, x_n; \theta) = \phi\left(w_0 + w_1x_1 + w_2x_2 + \cdots + w_nx_n\right), \tag{6.19}$$

where ϕ is the nonlinear activation function, and the set $\theta = \{w_0, w_1, \ldots, w_n\}$ represents the neuron's internal parameters.

In principle, ϕ can be any nonlinear function. Originally, the Heaviside step function

$$\phi(\alpha) = \begin{cases} 0, & \alpha < 0 \\ 1, & \alpha \geq 0 \end{cases} \tag{6.20}$$

was used as activation since biological neurons were thought to act like a digital switch. As long as the input α falls below some activation threshold, the switch will remain off and the output is 0. Once the input goes above the threshold, the switch gets turned on, producing an output equal to 1. This modeling was compatible with the belief that a biological neuron would not communicate with other downstream neurons unless it got excited or activated by a large enough input coming through its dendrites.

As we discussed in Chap. 5, the flat and discontinuous shape of the Heaviside step function creates fatal problems when we try to optimize machine learning models involving this function using gradient descent. Luckily, replacing the Heaviside step function with its smooth approximation, i.e., the logistic sigmoid function

$$\phi(\alpha) = \frac{1}{1 + e^{-\alpha}}, \tag{6.21}$$

ameliorates these optimization problems. For this reason, until the beginning of the twenty first century, most neural network models used the logistic sigmoid function or its close relative, the hyperbolic tangent function

[2] Typically, a bias parameter w_0 is also included in this linear combination.

$$\phi(\alpha) = \frac{e^{2\alpha} - 1}{e^{2\alpha} + 1} \tag{6.22}$$

as activation. Still as can be seen in Fig. 6.5, both the logistic and hyperbolic tangent functions are almost flat when the input is far away from the origin. This means that the derivative is almost zero when the input happens to be somewhat large (in either positive or negative direction). This issue, sometimes referred to as the *vanishing gradient* problem, hinders proper parameter tuning and limits practical use of the activation functions in (6.21) and (6.22).

More recently, a new breed of nonlinear activation functions based on the rectified linear unit (ReLU) function

$$\phi(\alpha) = \max(0, \alpha) \tag{6.23}$$

has shown better optimization performance compared to the previous and more biologically plausible options. Notice that with the ReLU function in (6.23) the derivative never vanishes as long as the input remains positive (see the bottom-left panel of Fig. 6.5). However, negative inputs can still create problems. To remedy this issue, a variant of the original ReLU called the *leaky* ReLU

$$\phi(\alpha) = \begin{cases} 1, & \alpha \geq 0 \\ \tau\alpha, & \alpha < 0 \end{cases} \tag{6.24}$$

was introduced, wherein the left "hinge" is no longer flat, but at a small incline (see the bottom-middle panel of Fig. 6.5). Another popular variant of the ReLU is the so-called *maxout* activation function defined as

$$\phi(\alpha) = \max(\tau_1 + \tau_2\alpha, \tau_3 + \tau_4\alpha), \tag{6.25}$$

which takes the maximum of two linear combinations of the input. Empirically, artificial neural networks employing the maxout activation function have fewer technical issues during optimization and often converge faster to a solution. However, it has more internal parameters to tune. An instance of the maxout activation function is plotted in the last panel of Fig. 6.5.

Arranging several artificial neurons (like the one shown in Fig. 6.4) in a single column and connecting their respective outputs into another summation unit create a *single-layer neural network*, as illustrated in Fig. 6.6. Note that this is precisely the graphical representation of the model in (6.18), barring the bias parameter v_0. To avoid clutter in the figure, the parameters associated with the line segments connecting the inputs to the artificial neurons are stored in θ_1 through θ_m. Different settings of these parameters define distinct features. Hence, we can tune them together with the external parameters v_0 through v_m during model training and by minimizing an appropriate cost function depending on the problem at hand.

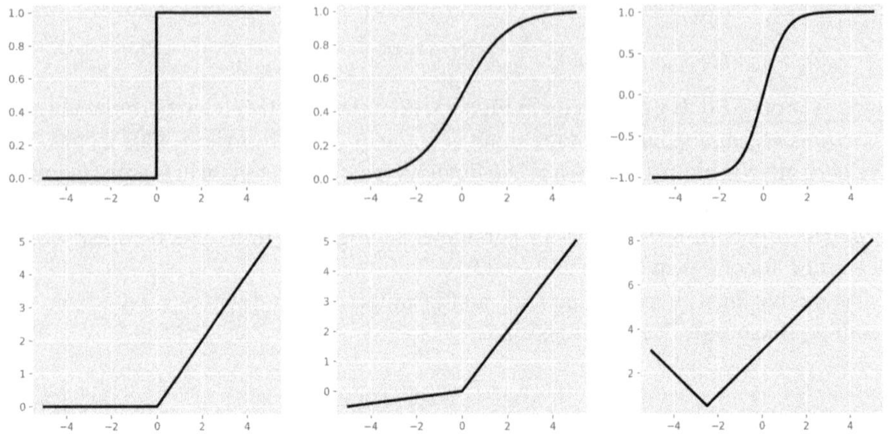

Fig. 6.5 An illustration of several historical and modern activation functions used in artificial neural networks. (Top-left panel) The Heaviside step function defined in (6.20). (Top-middle panel) The logistic sigmoid function defined in (6.21). (Top-right panel) The hyperbolic tangent function defined in (6.22). (Bottom-left panel) The rectified linear unit (ReLU) function defined in (6.23). (Bottom-middle panel) The leaky ReLU function defined in (6.24) with τ set to 0.1. (Bottom-right panel) The maxout activation function defined in (6.25) with $(\tau_1, \tau_2, \tau_3, \tau_4)$ set to $(3, 1, -2, -1)$

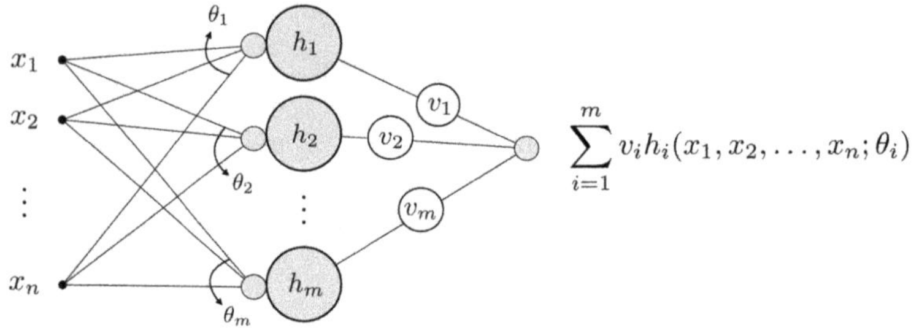

Fig. 6.6 A single-layer neural network illustrated

Multi-Layer Neural Networks

In this section, we study multi-layer perceptrons as a natural extension of single-layer neural networks introduced previously. Recall from Sect. "Feature Learning" and Fig. 6.6 therein that we built a single-layer neural network simply by taking multiple linear combinations of the inputs and passing each through a nonlinear activation function, and linearly combining the results. We can roughly summarize this process as

$$\text{linear combination} \rightarrow \text{nonlinear activation} \rightarrow \text{linear combination}. \tag{6.26}$$

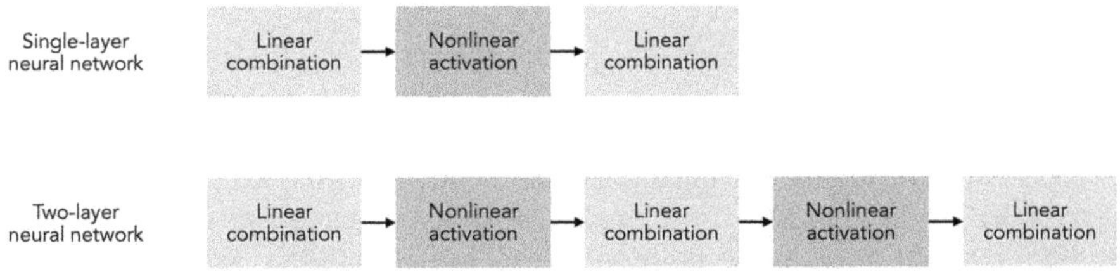

Fig. 6.7 A descriptive recipe for creating a single-layer neural network (top row) and a two-layer neural network (bottom row)

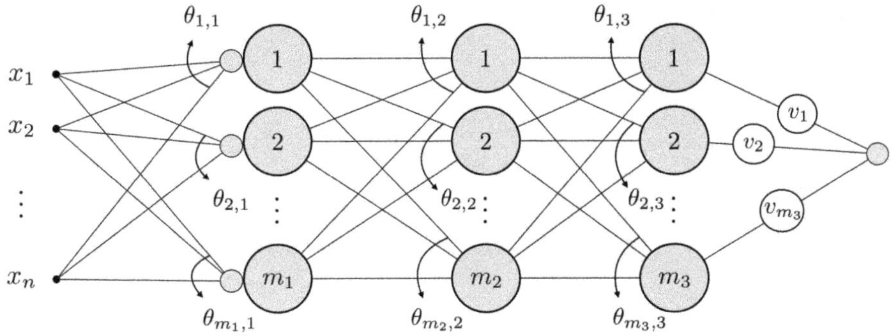

Fig. 6.8 A three-layer neural network illustrated. Note that the number of artificial neurons in each layer (denoted by m_1, m_2, and m_3) need not be the same

This is also illustrated in the top row of Fig. 6.7. Notice that nothing stops us from continuing this process further as depicted in the bottom row of Fig. 6.7, where the output of the single-layer neural network is passed through an extra pair of nonlinear activation and linear combination modules, creating a *two-layer neural network*. We can continue this process as many times as we wish to create a general multi-layer neural network, also known as a *multi-layer perceptron*. A neural network with several (typically more than three) layers is considered a *deep* network in the jargon of machine learning.

In Fig. 6.8, we show the graphical representation of a three-layer neural network that is analogous to the single-layer version shown in Fig. 6.6. Here, each of the three layers of artificial neurons separating the input layer on the left from the output on the right is called a *hidden* layer. The rationale behind this naming convention is that an outside observer can only "see" what goes inside the network (input) and what comes out of it (output), but not any intermediate layer in between.

Figure 6.8 also illustrates why multi-layer perceptrons are considered fully connected network architectures: because every unit in one layer is connected to every unit in the following layer. An important question to ask at this point is: how does using "deeper" neural networks benefit us? Let us explore this through a simple example.

Example 6.3 (From Shallow to Deep Neural Networks) In this example, we build a three-layer neural network using the hyperbolic tangent function as activation and initialize all the network's internal parameters at random. We then visually examine the outputs of several neurons from each layer of the network in Fig. 6.9. More specifically, we plot the outputs of four neurons from the first layer in the top row, four neurons from the second layer in the middle row, and four neurons from the third layer in the bottom row of Fig. 6.9. As expected, as we move from the top to the bottom of the figure (or from the shallow parts to the deeper parts of the network), the resulting functions take on a wider variety of shapes.

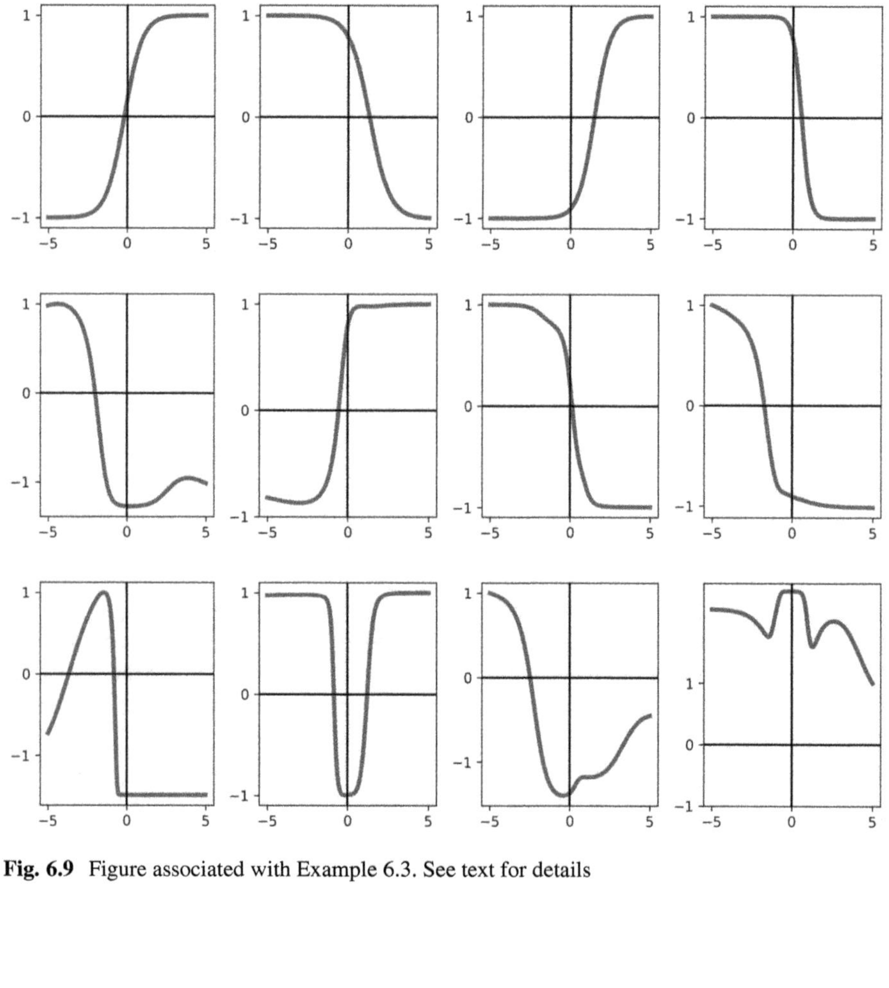

Fig. 6.9 Figure associated with Example 6.3. See text for details

Example 6.3 illustrates intuitively why deeper neural networks are superior to shallower ones: because they can represent much more complex nonlinear functions. This comes at a cost, however. Deep networks have more internal parameters and, generally speaking, are more difficult to optimize notwithstanding the fact that computation has become drastically faster and cheaper over the last decade. Next, we delve deeper into the optimization of deep neural networks.

Optimization of Neural Networks

While algorithms for minimizing neural network cost functions exist in a litany of forms, the vast majority of them are built upon a few principal foundations. First and foremost, these algorithms use the cost function's gradient just like the vanilla gradient descent algorithm introduced in Sect. "The Gradient Descent Algorithm" to minimize the cross-entropy cost for linear classification. In (5.34), we computed the gradient manually and in closed algebraic form. With neural networks, however, this becomes an extremely tedious task due to a large number of parameters involved as well as the compositional structure of these networks that requires the repeated use of the chain rule.[3]

Fortunately, by using a so-called *automatic differentiator*, it is possible to calculate gradients automatically and with ease, just as it is possible to multiply two large numbers using a conventional calculator. The inner-workings of an automatic differentiator are, for the most part, outside the scope of this book.[4] However, it is worthwhile to mention that a specific mode of automatic differentiation (the reverse mode, to be precise) is typically referred to as *backpropagation* in the machine learning literature. In other words, the backpropagation algorithm is the name given to the automatic computation of gradients for cost functions involving artificial neural networks.

Another common theme shared by most neural network optimizers is the use of gradient descent (or other optimizers) in "stochastic mode." In stochastic optimization, we do not use the entire training data in order to compute the gradient of the cost function. Notice, from (4.22) and (5.18), where the least squares cost for regression and the cross-entropy cost for classification are defined, that in both cases the cost function can be decomposed over individual data points. In other words, we can write a generic regression or classification cost function $g(\mathbf{w})$ as

---

[3] According to the chain rule, if we have $y = f_1(u)$ and $u = f_2(x)$, then the derivative of the composition of f_1 and f_2, i.e., $f_1(f_2(x))$, can be found as

$$\frac{\mathrm{d}y}{\mathrm{d}x} = \frac{\mathrm{d}y}{\mathrm{d}u} \times \frac{\mathrm{d}u}{\mathrm{d}x}.$$

[4] The interested reader is encouraged to see [3] and references therein.

$$g(\mathbf{w}) = \frac{1}{p}\sum_{i=1}^{p} g_i(\mathbf{w}), \tag{6.27}$$

where g_1 through g_p are individual cost functions associated with each of the p data points. To compute the gradient of g, we can write

$$\nabla g(\mathbf{w}) = \nabla\left(\frac{1}{p}\sum_{i=1}^{p} g_i(\mathbf{w})\right) = \frac{1}{p}\sum_{i=1}^{p} \nabla g_i(\mathbf{w}). \tag{6.28}$$

This means that the full (or batch) gradient is the summation of the gradients associated with each individual data point. Based on this observation, it is fair to ask what would happen if instead of taking one descent step in g using the full gradient, we took a sequence of p descent steps in $g_1, g_2, \ldots, g_p$ in a sequential manner. That is, we first descend in g_1 using $\nabla g_1(\mathbf{w})$, then in g_2 using $\nabla g_2(\mathbf{w})$, and so forth. It turns out that this approach provides faster convergence to the minima of g in practice.

In general, we can group multiple data points into a *mini-batch* and take a descent step in the cost function associated with the entire mini-batch. Suppose we partition the full training set $\{(\mathbf{x}_1, y_1), \ldots, (\mathbf{x}_p, y_p)\}$ into T non-overlapping subsets or mini-batches of roughly the same size, represented by Ω_1 through Ω_T. In this approach, we decompose the full gradient over each mini-batch as

$$\nabla g(\mathbf{w}) = \nabla\left(\frac{1}{p}\sum_{i=1}^{T}\sum_{j\in\Omega_i} g_j(\mathbf{w})\right) = \frac{1}{p}\sum_{i=1}^{T}\nabla\left(\sum_{j\in\Omega_i} g_j(\mathbf{w})\right) \tag{6.29}$$

and take descent steps sequentially, first in $\sum_{j\in\Omega_1} g_j(\mathbf{w})$, then in $\sum_{j\in\Omega_2} g_j(\mathbf{w})$, and so on. The optimal mini-batch size varies from problem to problem but in most cases is set relatively small compared to the full size of the training dataset. Note that with stochastic gradient descent the mini-batch size equals 1.

Design of Neural Network Architectures

As we discussed in Sect. "Multi-Layer Neural Networks", the larger the number of layers in a neural network, the higher its capacity to model complex nonlinear relationships. This suggests that when it comes to deciding the optimal number of layers in a neural network architecture, the more is the better, and we should make our networks as deep as possible until our computational resources run out. This seemingly logical conclusion, however, is not true. In the example below, we explore why this is the case.

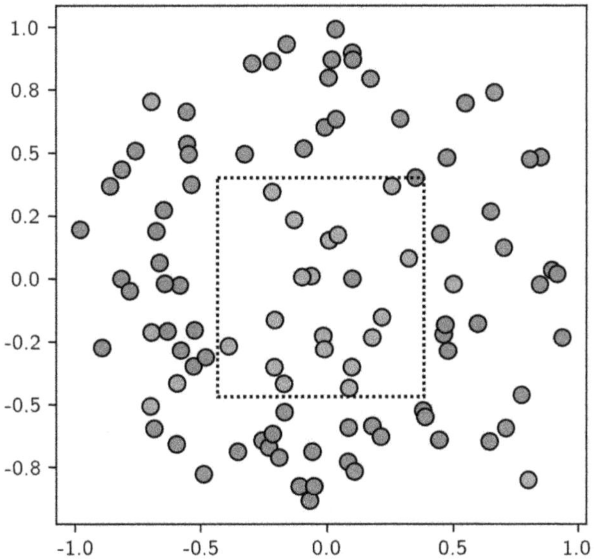

Fig. 6.10 A noisy two-class classification dataset

Example 6.4 (Classification Using Multi-layer Neural Networks) Figure 6.10 shows a simulated two-class classification dataset wherein the data points belonging to the "red" class (for the most part) fall within a rectangular region centered around the origin (highlighted by dashed boundaries). Notice that this dataset is *noisy* meaning that there are few "red" points that unexpectedly lie outside the small rectangular box, just as there is one "blue" point that falls inside the box surrounded by several "red" points. The existence of this level of noise is to be expected in any real-world classification dataset.

In Fig. 6.11, we show the result of classifying this data using three different neural network architectures. From left to right, these networks have one, two, and three hidden layers, respectively, each with the same number of artificial neurons per layer. Lacking adequate nonlinear capacity, the single-layer network leads to a large number of classification errors (left panel). The two-layer network seems to have recovered a decision boundary (middle panel) that resembles the true rectangular boundary shown in Fig. 6.10. Thanks to its abundant nonlinear capacity, the three-layer network learns a rather complex decision boundary (right panel) that classifies each data point "correctly" including the noisy ones.

As we saw in Example 6.4, increasing nonlinear capacity by adding more hidden layers to a neural network layer reduces the number of classification errors. However, the learned classification boundary tends to get worse—after a certain

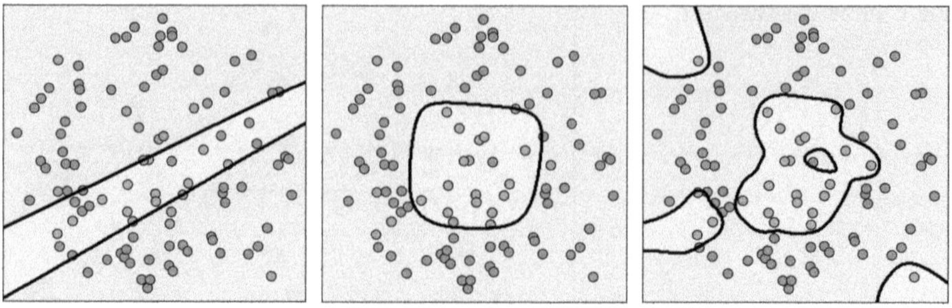

Fig. 6.11 Figure associated with Example 6.4. See text for further details

point—in terms of how it represents the underlying phenomenon that generated the classification data. The single-layer classification boundary shown in the left panel of Fig. 6.11 is an instance of a machine learning model that *underfits* the training data. This typically occurs because the chosen model does not have enough nonlinear capacity to capture the complexity of the underlying data. On the other hand, the three-layer classification boundary shown in the right panel of Fig. 6.11 is an instance of a model that *overfits* the training data. This occurs because the chosen model has too much nonlinear capacity that allows it to fit not only the signal but also the inevitable noise in the data. While such models fit the training data extremely well, they do so at the cost of not representing the underlying phenomenon well. The result is the models that perform extremely well in training, but fail spectacularly in testing or in deployment.

Diagnosing whether a machine model underfits or overfits the data is relatively easy. If, upon completion of parameter tuning, the training error remains high, then we can infer that the model underfits the data, in which case the nonlinear capacity of the model should be boosted (e.g., via adding more hidden layers). However, if the model performs well on the training set, we will not know whether it overfits the data until we evaluate it on a portion of the data that was not included as part of the training. It is therefore necessary to leave out a subset of the training data, commonly referred to as *validation* data, in order to validate the performance of the model for the purpose of diagnosing overfitting. An overfitting model will produce a (relatively) small training error but at the same time a (relatively) large validation error.

There is no precise rule for what portion of the training data should be set aside for validation. As a general rule of thumb, the larger the training data, the larger the fraction that can be saved for validation. When data is plenty, this fraction can be as large as $\frac{1}{2}$. When dealing with smaller datasets, however, the model should not be deprived of so much valuable training data. In such cases, we can randomly split the training data into k non-overlapping subsets or folds. Next, we leave out one of the folds for validation and combine the remaining $k-1$ folds for training. This way, $\frac{k-1}{k}$ of the original data will be used for training. We repeat this process k times, each time using a different fold for validation, averaging the resulting k

validation errors in the end. This validation scheme, commonly known as *k-fold cross-validation*, allows the model to use a larger share of the data in exchange for increased computation. In general, the smaller the data the larger k should be set. In most extreme cases when the data is severely limited, it is recommended to set k to its maximum possible value (i.e., the number of points in the training set). By doing so, we will leave only one data point out at a time for validation. This particular setting is called *leave-one-out* cross-validation.

Cross-validation provides a way to answer the question we posed in the beginning of this section: how should we choose the right number of hidden layers to include in a neural network model? In short, to design a well-performing neural network architecture for use with a given dataset, we cross-validate an array of choices, selecting the model that results in the lowest cross-validation error. It is important to remember that in building a neural network architecture, our design choices, in addition to the network's depth, include the number of artificial neurons per layer as well as the nonlinear form of the activation function.

Problems

6.1 Completing Example 6.1

In Example 6.1, we examined the growth pattern of a bacterial species over time and engineered a logistic feature that linearized the originally nonlinear dataset provided in Table 6.1. Use the proposed feature in (6.13) and train a linear regression model (as described in Chap. 4) for the linearized version of the data shown in the right panel of Fig. 6.1. Then, rewrite the learned model as a function of the original input and plot it in the original space of the problem (shown in the left panel of Fig. 6.1).

6.2 Nonlinear Feature Engineering for Regression

A simulated regression dataset consisting of $p = 16$ input–output pairs is provided in Table 6.2 and plotted in Fig. 6.12. Use your knowledge of mathematical functions and operations from Chap. 3 to engineer a proper nonlinear feature that could linearize this dataset. You should then transform the input using your engineered feature and solve the resulting linear regression problem. Finally, plot the learned regressor in both the original and feature space of the problem.

6.3 Feature Engineering vs. Feature Learning

Compare the feature engineering and feature learning paradigms in terms of (i) model performance and (ii) computation. Does one paradigm have a better chance of improving performance than the other? Which paradigm requires more computational resources and why?

6.4 ReLUs for the Win

In Sect. "Feature Learning", we introduced a host of old and modern activation functions used in the design of artificial neural networks. Describe why the

Table 6.2 Data associated with Exercise 6.2

Input x	Output y
0.96	1.28
0.46	2.47
0.39	3.11
0.48	2.17
0.11	3.42
0.09	2.92
0.72	−0.04
0.66	0.48
0.61	0.63
0.76	−0.05
0.41	3.1
0.58	0.95
0.88	0.48
0.23	3.95
0.94	1.23
0.12	3.44

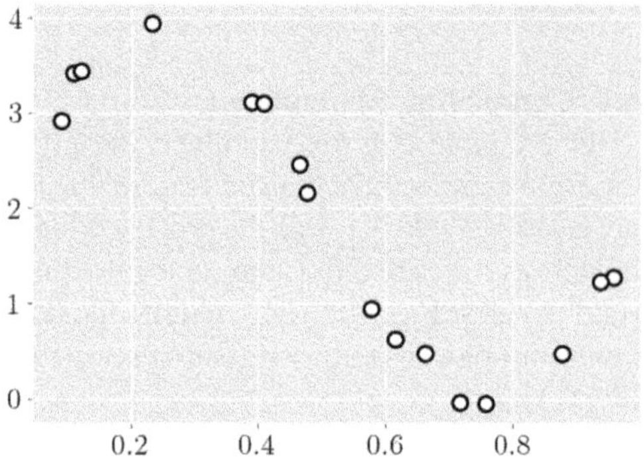

Fig. 6.12 Figure associated with Exercise 6.2

activation functions based on the rectified linear unit (ReLU) have largely replaced the older ones?

6.5 Counting the Parameters of a Multi-layer Neural Network

(a) Find the total number of adjustable parameters in the single-layer neural network displayed in Fig. 6.6. Express your answer in terms of the dimension of the input n and the number of artificial neurons m in the network's only hidden layer.
(b) Find the total number of adjustable parameters in the three-layer neural network displayed in Fig. 6.8. Express your answer in terms of the dimension of the input n and the number of artificial neurons in each hidden layer, i.e., m_1, m_2, and m_3.
(c) Using your answers to part (a) and part (b), find a general formula for computing the total number of adjustable parameters in an ℓ-layer neural network. Once

again, express your answer in terms of the dimension of the input n as well as the number of artificial neurons in each hidden layer.

6.6 Backpropagation for a Single-Layer Neural Network

Compute the gradient of a cross-entropy cost function associated with a single-layer neural network. The cross-entropy cost function is defined in (5.31). For simplicity, assume the hidden layer of the network consists only of two artificial neurons.

6.7 Backpropagation for a Two-Layer Neural Network

Compute the gradient of a least squares cost function associated with a two-layer neural network. The least squares cost function is defined in (4.22). For simplicity, assume both hidden layers of the network consist only of two artificial neurons each.

References

1. Lin J, Lee SM, Lee HJ, Koo YM. Modeling of typical microbial cell growth in batch culture. Biotechnol Bioprocess Eng. 2000;5(5):382–85
2. Borhani S, Borhani R, Kajdacsy-Balla A. Artificial intelligence: a promising frontier in bladder cancer diagnosis and outcome prediction. Crit Rev Oncol Hematol. 2022;171:103601. https://doi.org/10.1016/j.critrevonc.2022.103601
3. Watt J, Borhani R, Katsaggelos AK. Machine learning refined: foundations, algorithms, and applications. Cambridge: Cambridge University Press; 2020

Chapter 7
Convolutional and Recurrent Neural Networks

As we saw in the previous chapter, artificial neural networks (and more precisely single- and multi-layer perceptrons) are powerful tools for modeling nonlinear input–output relationships. For instance, we may seek to uncover the relationship between a patient's lab test results (input) and the likelihood of readmission to hospital in near future (output)—if such relationship exists—using a single-layer perceptron model like the one shown in Fig. 7.1. It is important to note that such a model is not sensitive to the order in which the input is fed to it. Here, the first four inputs are liver function test results, and the next four are urine test results. If we switched this around and fed the urine test results first (as inputs 1 through 4) and the liver function test results last (as inputs 5 through 8), nothing would fundamentally change with respect to the underlying model that would be trained using this data. In fact, with fully connected perceptrons, there is no such thing as the first input versus the last input since the order here is completely arbitrary.

This, however, is not always the case. Sometimes, the input data will have some sort of structure that can—and should—be leveraged when solving machine learning and deep learning problems involving that data type. In other words, we cannot simply switch the input around and expect the model to perform equally well. Images and texts are prime examples of such type of data.

As discussed in Sect. "Imaging Data", the information in an image is stored over a rectangular grid (matrix) at small square units (entries) called pixels. The pixel values alone are, for the most part, of little to no use without knowledge of their exact location on the grid. To see why this is the case, compare the two images shown in Fig. 7.2, wherein the image on the right has the exact same pixel values as the one on the left. By shuffling the pixels around, however, all the spatial

Supplementary Information The online version contains supplementary material available at https://doi.org/10.1007/978-3-031-19502-0_7.

R. Borhani et al., *Fundamentals of Machine Learning and Deep Learning in Medicine*, https://doi.org/10.1007/978-3-031-19502-0_7

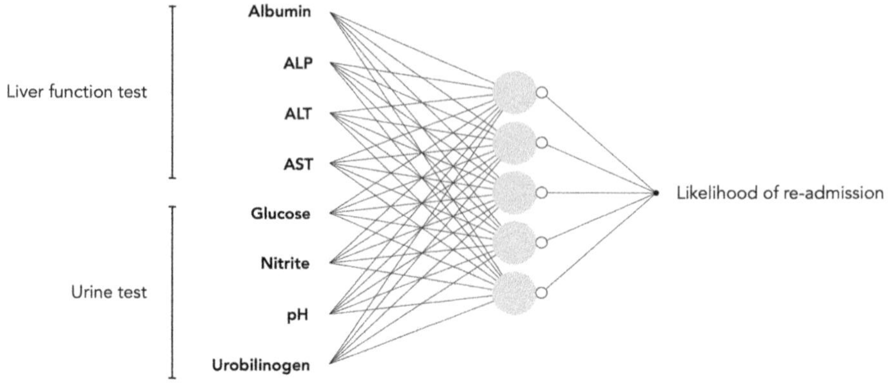

Fig. 7.1 A single-layer perceptron that takes as input four liver function test results (albumin, ALP, ALT, and AST levels) and four urine test results (glucose, nitrite, pH, and urobilinogen levels), and outputs the likelihood of the patient's readmission to the hospital in the near future

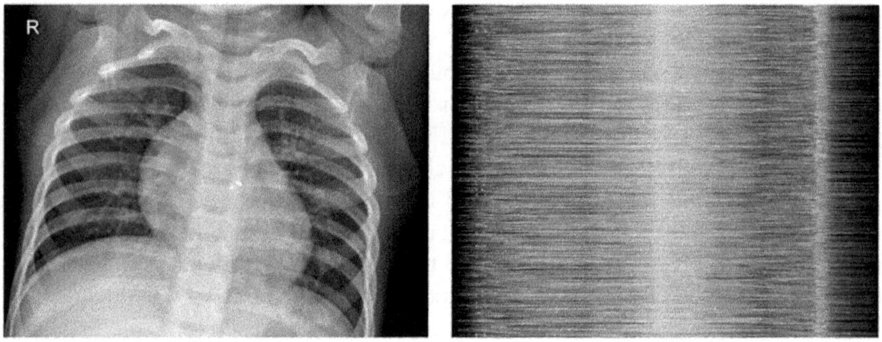

Fig. 7.2 The image in the right panel was created by a random shuffling of the rows in the original X-ray on the left. While the two images share the exact same pixel values, virtually all the useful medical information in the original image is lost after altering spatial placement of the pixels

information encoded in the original image is lost, and the resulting scrambled image looks nothing like the original, despite having the exact same pixel values.

Similarly, text data (as well as a host of other data types such as genome-sequencing data, time-series data, etc.) possess a special sequential structure that must not be ignored during modeling. For example, a physician instruction note that reads "take 40 mg omeprazole before breakfast and 10 mg atorvastatin at night" would completely lose its meaning if we were to shuffle the words in it at random (see the top panel of Fig. 7.3), or worse, would take on an intelligible but different meaning that could be detrimental to the patient's health (see the bottom panel of Fig. 7.3).

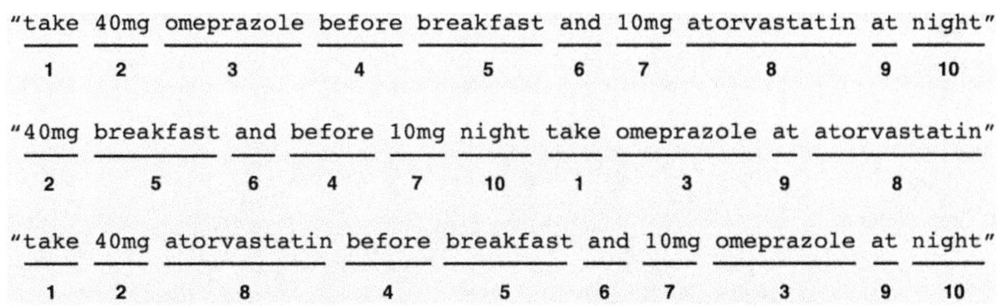

Fig. 7.3 Different word permutations of a physician note instructing the patient to take two medications: one over-the-counter drug for acid reflux (omeprazole), and one prescribed medication for high cholesterol (atrovastatin). While the scrambled version in the middle row is unintelligible, the permutation in the bottom row changes the meaning of the original order that can be harmful to the patient

For the reasons detailed above, generic multi-layer perceptrons are not suitable for modeling imaging and text data. In this chapter, we discuss two popular neural network architectures that are designed respectively to handle imaging and text data as input, namely, convolutional neural networks and recurrent neural networks.

The Convolution Operation

In Sect. "Time-Series Data", we introduced time-series data as a one-dimensional data type that is commonly used in machine learning. Figure 7.4 shows a time-series dataset depicting the daily number of new cases of Covid-19 in Cook County, Illinois, collected over a 1-year period starting from June 1, 2020, through June 1, 2021. As can be seen in the figure, the time-series data fluctuates rather rapidly from one day to the next, giving it an overall "jagged" appearance. Most, if not all, time-series datasets exhibit some amount of jaggedness that is typically attributed to the presence of high-frequency (or rapidly changing) noise perturbing the underlying low-frequency (or smooth) signal.

For example, the sharp spike seen in Fig. 7.4 on November 1, 2020 was most likely created as a result of a delay in reporting the number of cases from the day before (notice that 0 cases were reported on the last day of October 2020). One quick way to fix this (type of) error would be to keep only half of the number of reported cases on November 1 and assign the remaining half to the prior day.[1] In general, it is not always easy to identify the source of error/noise in a time-series data (as we did here).

---

[1] A similar reporting error seems to have happened on January 1, 2021.

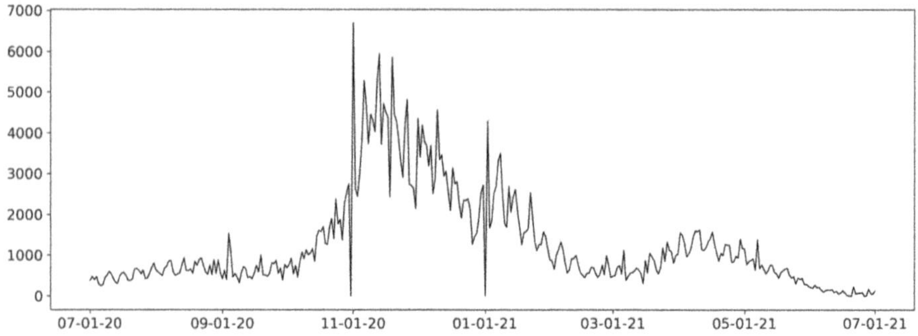

Fig. 7.4 The daily number of new cases of Covid-19 in Cook County, Illinois, as reported by the New York Times [1]

Denoising—or the automatic removal of noise from observed data—is a classical problem in signal processing. In the context of time-series analysis, denoising is generally performed as a preprocessing step in order to improve our understanding and summarization of overall trends in the data. As we will soon see, the convolution operation arises naturally as one way to solve the denoising problem.

To state the problem formally, we assume the observed data x to be made up of two components: a signal component s and a noise component ε. Therefore, the N data points in the time-series $x_1, x_2, \ldots, x_N$ can be decomposed and written as

$$\begin{aligned} x_1 &= s_1 + \varepsilon_1, \\ x_2 &= s_2 + \varepsilon_2, \\ &\vdots \\ x_N &= s_N + \varepsilon_N. \end{aligned} \tag{7.1}$$

To recover the signal s from the observation x, we make two reasonably realistic assumptions: one that the noise ε has no bias (and thus has zero mean) and two that the underlying signal s is relatively smooth. The latter is sometimes called the *local smoothness* assumption in the jargon of machine learning. This assumption is valid in the case of the Covid time-series data in Fig. 7.4 because in the absence of noise we should expect that the number of new Covid cases in one region (Cook County) to not change drastically from one day to the next.

According to (7.1), the average of all observed data in an L-vicinity of x_n (i.e., the $2L+1$ consecutive data points $x_{n-L},\ x_{n-L+1},\ \ldots,\ x_n,\ \ldots,\ x_{n+L-1},\ x_{n+L}$) can be written as

$$\frac{1}{2L+1}\sum_{\ell=-L}^{L} x_{n+\ell} = \frac{1}{2L+1}\sum_{\ell=-L}^{L} s_{n+\ell} + \frac{1}{2L+1}\sum_{\ell=-L}^{L} \varepsilon_{n+\ell}. \tag{7.2}$$

Now, leveraging our first assumption that ε has zero mean, we can write

$$\frac{1}{2L+1}\sum_{\ell=-L}^{L} \varepsilon_{n+\ell} \approx 0. \tag{7.3}$$

Next, using our second assumption that s is smooth, we can write

$$\frac{1}{2L+1}\sum_{\ell=-L}^{L} s_{n+\ell} \approx s_n. \tag{7.4}$$

Finally, substituting (7.3) and (7.4) into (7.2), we arrive at the following estimation for the value of s_n

$$s_n \approx \frac{1}{2L+1}\sum_{\ell=-L}^{L} x_{n+\ell}. \tag{7.5}$$

Statistically speaking, the larger the value of L the more reliable the approximation in (7.3) becomes, as more samples generally drive the "sample average" closer to the "population average" (which is assumed to be zero). On the other hand, as L gets larger, the approximation in (7.4) gets worse, as s_n gets drowned out by its neighboring values. Fortunately, we can ameliorate this issue by adjusting the way we compute the average in (7.5). Specifically, rather than using a *uniform* average, we take a *weighted* average of elements in the L-vicinity of x_n such that larger weights are assigned to the elements closer to x_n and smaller weights to those farther away from it.

Denoting by w_ℓ the weight given to $x_{n+\ell}$ in (7.5), we can write it more generally as

$$s_n = \sum_{\ell=-L}^{L} w_\ell \, x_{n+\ell}, \tag{7.6}$$

where we have also replaced the "approximately equal" sign with its strict version. Notice that (7.6) reduces to (7.5) when the weights are chosen uniformly, as

$$w_\ell = \frac{1}{2L+1}, \qquad \ell = -L, \ldots, L. \tag{7.7}$$

Figure 7.5 shows a graphical illustration of the uniform weight sequence in (7.7) as well as the non-uniform weight sequence defined entry-wise as

$$w_\ell = \frac{L+1-|\ell|}{(L+1)^2}, \qquad \ell = -L, \ldots, L. \tag{7.8}$$

Note that the non-uniform weight sequence in (7.8) attains its maximum value when $\ell = 0$ (this is the weight assigned to x_n). The weights then taper off gradually as we get farther away from the center point at x_n. Note, also, that the weights in both (7.7) and (7.8) always add up to 1.

The term *convolution* refers to the weighted sum in (7.6). More precisely, the convolution between w (a sequence of length $2L + 1$ defined over the range $-L, \ldots, L$) and x (a sequence of length N defined over the range $1, \ldots, N$) is a new sequence s denoted by $s = w * x$, and defined entry-wise as[2]

$$s_n = \sum_{\ell=-L}^{L} w_\ell \, x_{n+\ell} \qquad n = 1, 2, \ldots, N. \tag{7.10}$$

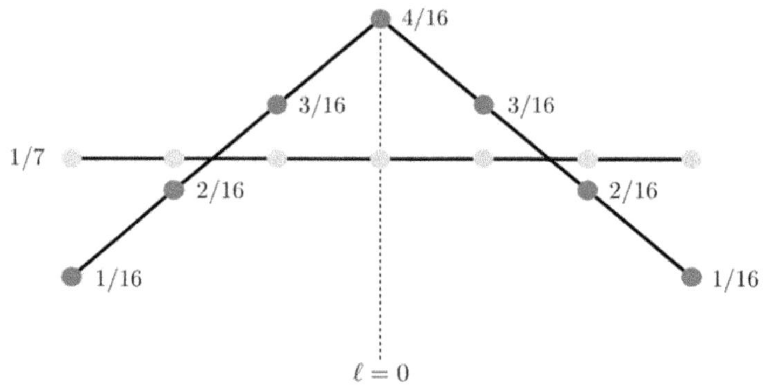

Fig. 7.5 An illustration of two weighting schemes: uniform (in yellow) as defined in (7.7) and non-uniform (in blue) as defined in (7.8). In both cases, $L = 3$

[2] The operation defined in (7.10) is more accurately known as *cross-correlation*, which is closely related to the convolution operation defined as

$$s_n = \sum_{\ell=-L}^{L} w_{-\ell} \, x_{n+\ell}, \tag{7.9}$$

where the weight sequence w is first flipped around its center before getting multiplied by x. Flipping the weight sequence guarantees the convolution operation to have the commutative property, which is not a matter of concern to us in this book. Therefore, with slight abuse of terminology, we continue to refer to the operation defined in (7.10) as convolution throughout the chapter.

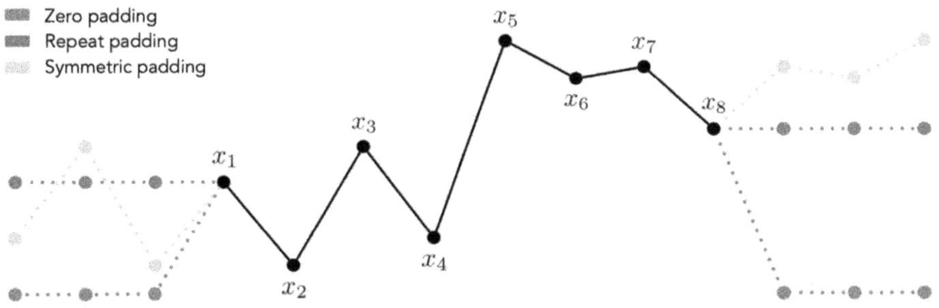

Fig. 7.6 An illustration of padding the sequence x (originally of length $N = 8$) with $L = 3$ elements on both sides, using zero padding (in red), repeat padding (in blue), and symmetric padding (in yellow)

The weight sequence w is sometimes referred to as the convolution *filter* or *kernel.* This is not to be confused with the term kernel used in other machine learning contexts (e.g., the kernel trick).

It is important to note that in order to compute the first entry of the convolution sequence using the definition in (7.10), we need to access some elements of x that do not exist! In other words, to compute s_1, we need the values of $x_{-L+1}, x_{-L+2}, \ldots, x_0$ that fall outside the original range of x. Similarly, the value of s_N depends on $x_{N+1}, x_{N+2}, \ldots, x_{N+L}$ that are undefined.

To fix this issue, we must add L entries to both the beginning and end of x, so that for every $1 \leq n \leq N$ the sequence x can be defined in an L-vicinity of x_n. This insertion operation is commonly referred to as *padding*. How we choose to pad x is—for the most part—inconsequential, particularly when L is much smaller than N (since padding only affects the first and last L elements of the resulting convolution s).

Figure 7.6 illustrates three common ways to pad x: (i) *zero padding*, where the input x is padded with zeros on both sides, (ii) *repeat padding*, where x is padded with the value of x_1 on the left, and with the value of x_N on the right, and (iii) *symmetric padding*, where x is mirrored around x_1 on the left, and x_N on the right.

Example 7.1 (Denoising the Covid-19 Time-Series Data) In this example, we use the convolution operation defined in (7.10) to denoise the Covid-19 time-series data plotted originally in Fig. 7.4. In Fig. 7.7, we show the results of convolving the input x with the weight kernel w defined in (7.8) for different values of L. Notice that as we increase the length of the convolutional kernel, the recovered signal (shown in red) becomes smoother.

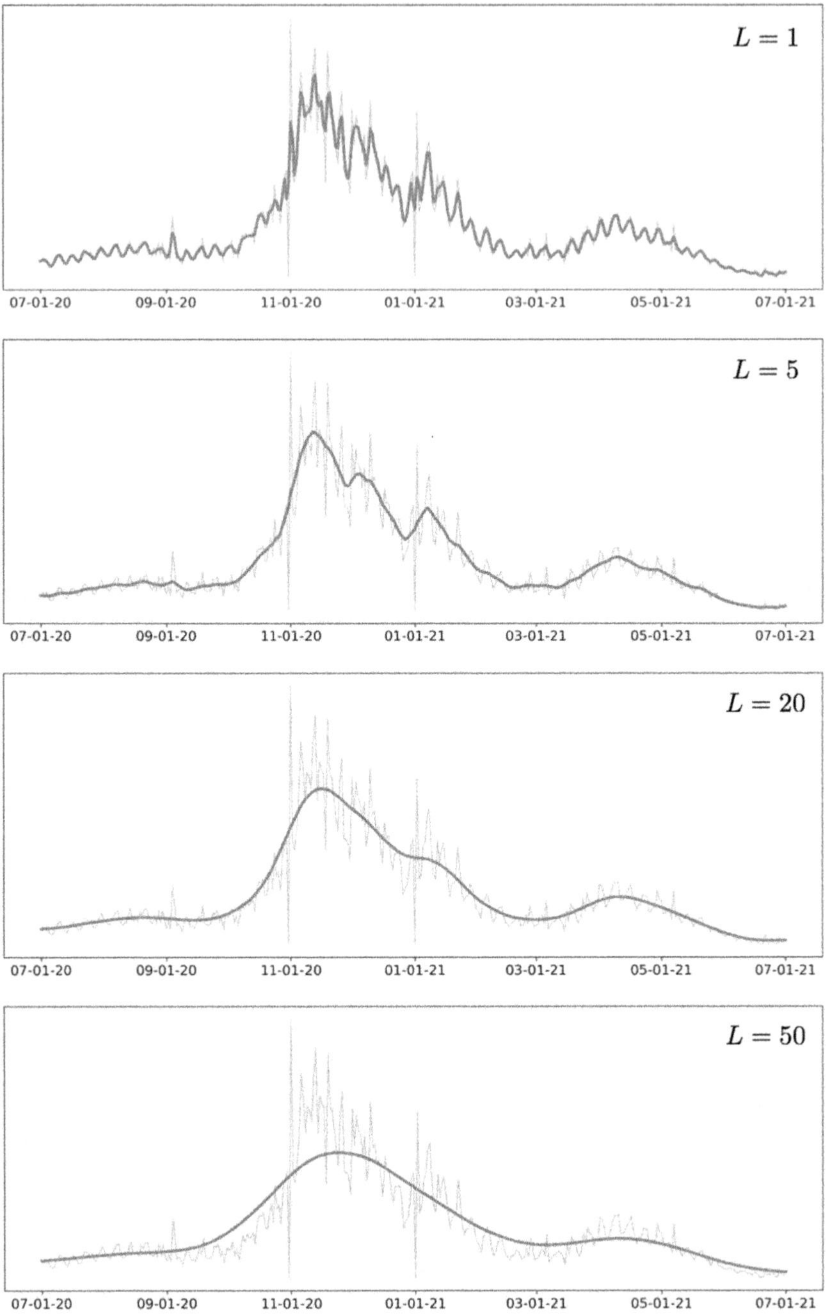

Fig. 7.7 Figure associated with Example 7.1. See text for details

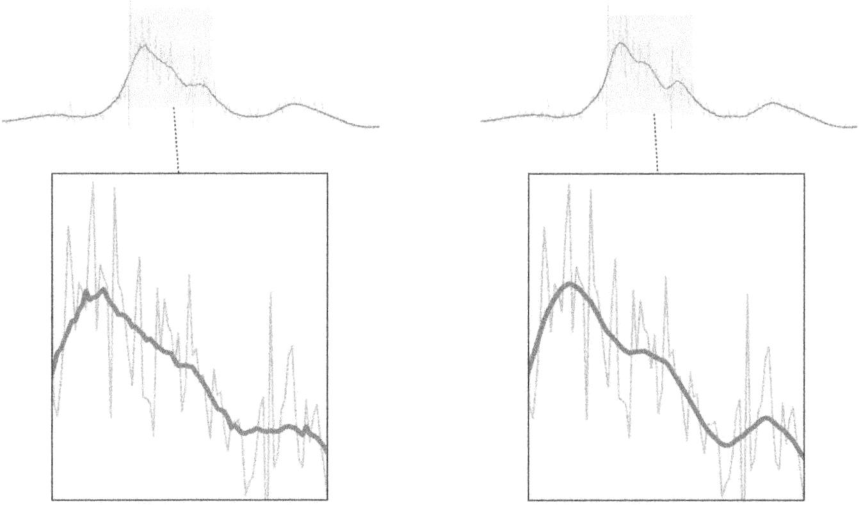

Fig. 7.8 Figure associated with Example 7.2. (Left panel) The convolution of the underlying time-series data (in gray) with the uniform kernel in (7.7). (Right panel) The convolution of the time-series data with the non-uniform kernel in (7.8). In both cases $L = 10$

Example 7.2 (Uniform Versus Non-uniform Convolutional Kernels) In this example, we examine how changing the weighting scheme of the convolutional kernel affects the shape of the recovered signal in the case of the Covid-19 time-series data in Fig. 7.4. Specifically, we convolve this data with both the uniform and non-uniform weight sequences defined in (7.7) and (7.8), respectively, and compare the results in Fig. 7.8. As you can see, the non-uniform scheme results in a much smoother recovery of the signal compared to the uniform one.

The convolution operation defined for one-dimensional sequences in (7.10) can be extended in a straightforward manner to higher dimensions. Here, we are particularly interested in the two-dimensional case where the convolution between w and x (denoted by $s = w * x$) is written entry-wise as

$$s_{n_1,n_2} = \sum_{\ell_1=-L_1}^{L_1} \sum_{\ell_2=-L_2}^{L_2} w_{\ell_1,\ell_2}\, x_{n_1+\ell_1,\, n_2+\ell_2} \qquad \begin{array}{l} n_1 = 1, 2, \ldots, N_1 \\ n_2 = 1, 2, \ldots, N_2 \end{array}, \tag{7.11}$$

where w is an $(2L_1 + 1) \times (2L_2 + 1)$ kernel matrix and x—which was an $N_1 \times N_2$ matrix originally—has been *padded* (e.g., with zeros) to become

(continued)

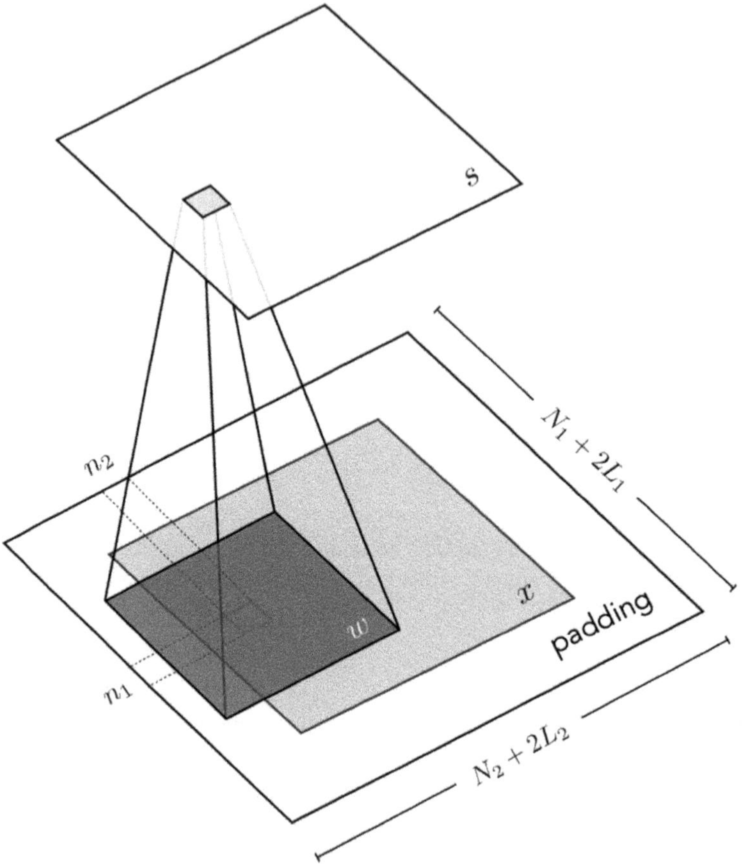

Fig. 7.9 An illustration of two-dimensional convolution. The convolutional kernel w (shown in blue) slides over the (padded) input x, performing an entry-wise multiplication with the part of the image it is currently placed on and then adding up the results into a single output pixel (shown in yellow). This process is repeated for every location in x, forming the matrix $s = w * x$

Example 7.2 (continued)
a matrix of size $(N_1 + 2L_1) \times (N_2 + 2L_2)$, so that s_{n_1,n_2} is defined for all $n_1 = 1, 2, \ldots, N_1$ and $n_2 = 1, 2, \ldots, N_2$.

Two-dimensional convolution is illustrated conceptually in Fig. 7.9. To compute s_{n_1,n_2} (shown in yellow), the convolutional kernel w (shown in navy blue) is placed on top of x, centered around the same location in x: that is, x_{n_1,n_2}. The sum of the entry-wise product between w and the portion of x it overlaps with is the resulting value for s_{n_1,n_2}.

Example 7.3 (Using Two-Dimensional Convolution to Find Image Gradients) Recall from our discussion in Example 3.3 that a grayscale image can be thought of as a function with two inputs and one output: the first input is a row number, the second input a column number, and the output is the intensity value of the pixel whose location in the image is dictated by the two inputs. Digital images, however, are not differentiable functions. In other words, we cannot simply use the limit

$$\frac{1}{2\epsilon}\begin{bmatrix} x\,(n_1+\epsilon,\, n_2) - x\,(n_1-\epsilon,\, n_2) \\ x\,(n_1,\, n_2+\epsilon) - x\,(n_1,\, n_2-\epsilon) \end{bmatrix} \tag{7.12}$$

in order to define the gradient of image x at point $(n_1,\, n_2)$ by sending $\epsilon \to 0$. This is the case because ϵ cannot be made arbitrarily small due to the discrete nature of the input. The best we can do is approximate the gradient in (7.12) by setting ϵ to the smallest valid value possible (in this case $\epsilon = 1$), giving the approximate image gradient as

$$\frac{1}{2}\begin{bmatrix} x\,(n_1+1,\, n_2) - x\,(n_1-1,\, n_2) \\ x\,(n_1,\, n_2+1) - x\,(n_1,\, n_2-1) \end{bmatrix} \tag{7.13}$$

or, equivalently using our subscript notation, as

$$\frac{1}{2}\begin{bmatrix} x_{n_1+1,\, n_2} - x_{n_1-1,\, n_2} \\ x_{n_1,\, n_2+1} - x_{n_1,\, n_2-1} \end{bmatrix}. \tag{7.14}$$

Each element of the image gradient in (7.14) can be written as a convolution between the image x and a certain convolutional kernel. More specifically, we can write

$$\frac{1}{2}\begin{bmatrix} x_{n_1+1,\, n_2} - x_{n_1-1,\, n_2} \\ x_{n_1,\, n_2+1} - x_{n_1,\, n_2-1} \end{bmatrix} = \begin{bmatrix} w_h * x \\ w_v * x \end{bmatrix}, \tag{7.15}$$

where

$$w_h = \begin{bmatrix} -0.5 & 0 & +0.5 \end{bmatrix} \tag{7.16}$$

and

$$w_v = \begin{bmatrix} -0.5 \\ 0 \\ +0.5 \end{bmatrix}. \tag{7.17}$$

(continued)

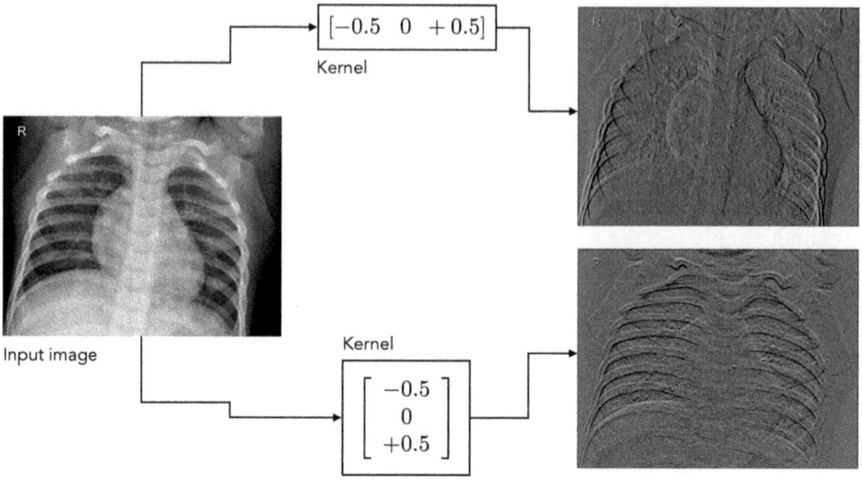

Fig. 7.10 Figure associated with Example 7.3. See text for details

Example 7.3 (continued)

In Fig. 7.10, we show the results of convolving an input image with the horizontal and vertical convolutional kernels in (7.16) and (7.16), respectively. The resulting images in this case have undergone contrast normalization for enhanced visualization.

Convolutional Neural Networks

Using individual raw pixel values as features has been shown experimentally to produce low-quality results in virtually all machine learning tasks involving images. Moreover, if were to use pixel values directly as features, high-resolution medical images of today would create ultra-high-dimensional feature spaces that are prone to a negative phenomenon in machine learning called *the curse of dimensionality* (see Sect. "Revisiting Feature Design" for a refresher).

An alternative, more efficient approach is to represent an image using its edge content alone. This idea is illustrated in Fig. 7.11 that shows an input image in the left panel along with a corresponding image in the right panel, comprised only of the most prominent edges in the original image.

The edge-detected image in the right panel of Fig. 7.11 is an efficient representation of the original image in the left panel in the sense that we can still—for the most part—tell what goes on inside the image while discarding a large amount of less-useful information from the vast majority of pixels that do not belong to any edges.

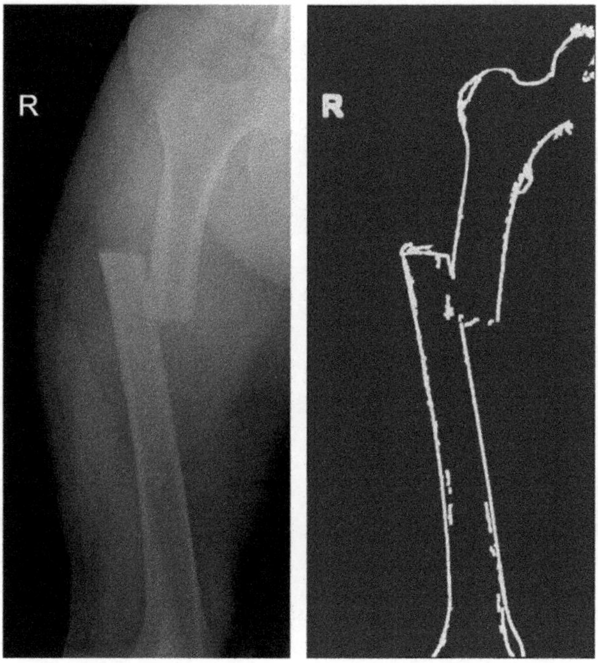

Fig. 7.11 (Left panel) An X-ray, taken from [2], showing a right femur chalk stick fracture. (Right panel) The edge-detected version of this image where the bright yellow pixels indicate large edge content

This is true in general: the most relevant visual information in an image is largely contained in the relatively small number of edges within the image [3]. Interestingly, several studies performed on mammals have also determined that individual neurons involved in early stages of visual processing operate as edge detectors [4, 5]. In computer vision, edge-based feature design has been the cornerstone of many popular feature engineering schemes including the histogram of oriented gradients (or HoG) [6] and the scale-invariant feature transform (or SIFT) [7].

The edges within an image can be extracted using the convolution operation. As illustrated in Fig. 7.10, convolving an image with certain horizontal and vertical kernels gives image gradients in those directions where large pixel values indicate strong edge content. Additional convolutional kernels may be added to the mix to detect edges that are not strictly horizontal or vertical but are at an incline. For example, each of the eight convolutional kernels shown in Fig. 7.12 corresponds to one of eight equally (angularly) spaced edge orientations starting from 0°, with seven additional orientations at 45° (or $\frac{\pi}{4}$-radian) increments.

To capture the total edge content of an input image in any of the eight directions shown in Fig. 7.12, we convolve the input image with the corresponding convolutional kernel, pass the results through a rectified linear unit (ReLU)

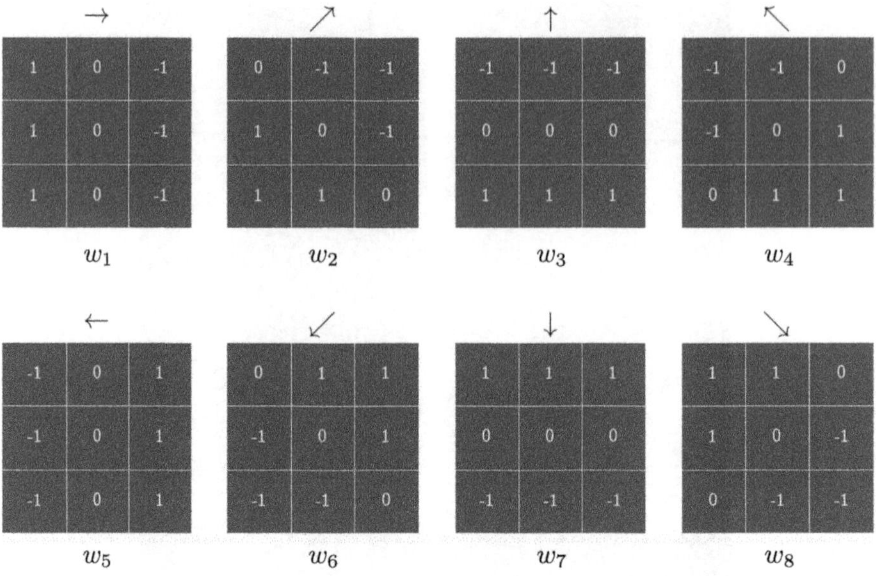

Fig. 7.12 Eight 3 × 3 convolutional kernels designed to detect horizontal, vertical, and diagonal edges within an image

function[3] to remove any negative entries, and finally add up the remaining pixel values into a single scalar. Denoting the input image by x, and the convolutional kernels by $w_1, w_2, \ldots, w_8$, this edge extraction process returns eight feature maps $f_1, f_2, \ldots, f_8$ to represent x, which can be expressed algebraically as

$$f_i = \sum_{\text{all pixels}} \max(0,\ w_i * x) \qquad i = 1, 2, \ldots, 8. \tag{7.18}$$

We use the ReLU function in (7.18) so that negative values in the matrix $w_i * x$ do not cancel out positive values in it when performing the final summation.[4]

Stacking all f_i's into a single vector $\mathbf{f}$, we now have a (primitive) feature representation for x in the form of a histogram which can be normalized to have unit length.[5]

[3] See Sect. "Min–Max Operations" for a refresher on the ReLU function.

[4] Note that we are not discarding any information by removing negative entries in $w_i * x$ since those entries are precisely the positive entries present in $w_j * x$ when $|i - j| = 4$ and vice versa (see Fig. 7.12).

[5] This can be done by dividing each entry in the vector $\mathbf{f}$ by the vector's norm, i.e.,

$$\mathbf{f} \leftarrow \frac{\mathbf{f}}{\|\mathbf{f}\|}.$$

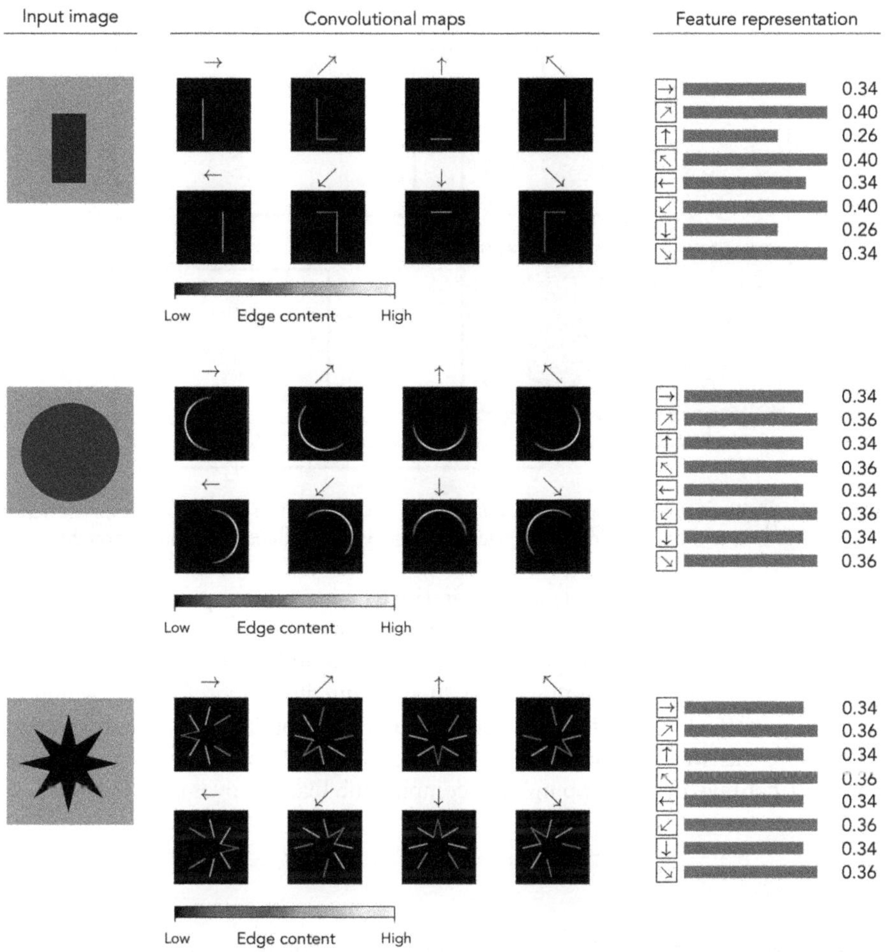

Fig. 7.13 An illustration of a simple edge-based feature representation based on (7.18). See text for further details

This feature extraction process is illustrated in Fig. 7.13 for three simple images: a rectangle (top panel), a circle (middle panel), and an eight-angled star or octagram (bottom panel). For each basic shape, we plot the convolutional maps of the input image with each of the eight kernels in Fig. 7.12 (after passing each map through ReLU), as well as the final histogram representation of the image in the last column.

The edge-based feature extractor we have designed so far works well in overly simplistic cases. For example, we can distinguish an image of a circle from that of a square by simply comparing their feature representations. As can be seen in Fig. 7.13, the feature representation of a circle is much more uniform than (and thus distinct from) that of a square. This strategy, however, fails when applied to

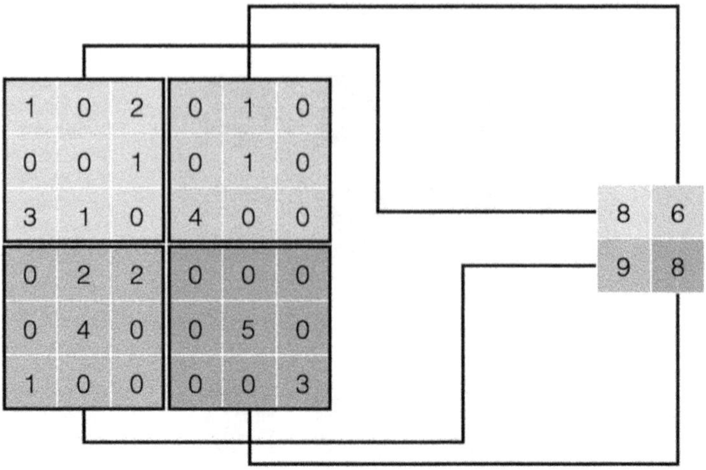

Fig. 7.14 An illustration of the summation pooling operation. The 6×6 matrix on the left is pooled over four non-overlapping 3×3 patches, producing the smaller 2×2 matrix on the right

distinguishing between a circle and a star, since their feature representations end up to be identical due to the symmetrical nature of both shapes.

In practice, real-world images are much more complicated than these simplistic geometrical shapes, and summarizing them using just eight features would be extremely ineffective. To fix this issue, instead of computing each feature over the entire image as was done in (7.18), we break the image down into relatively small patches (that may be overlapping) and compute the features over each patch as

$$f_{i,j} = \sum_{j\text{th patch}} \max(0,\ w_i * x) \qquad i = 1, 2, \ldots, 8. \tag{7.19}$$

This process, that is, breaking the image into small (possibly overlapping) patches and representing each patch via the sum (or average) of its pixels, is referred to as *pooling* in the parlance of machine learning and is depicted in Fig. 7.14 for a sample 6×6 matrix.

Procedurally, the pooling operation is very similar to convolution but with two differences: first, with pooling the sliding window can jump multiple pixels at a time depending on how much overlap is required between adjacent windows or patches. The number of pixels the sliding window is shifted each time is usually referred to as the *stride*. With convolution, the stride is typically set to 1. The second difference between convolution and pooling is how the content of the sliding window is processed and then summarized as a single value. Recall that with convolution, we must first compute the entry-wise product between the kernel matrix and the matrix captured inside the sliding window. With pooling, however, there is no kernel involved, and we simply add up all the pixels inside the sliding window.

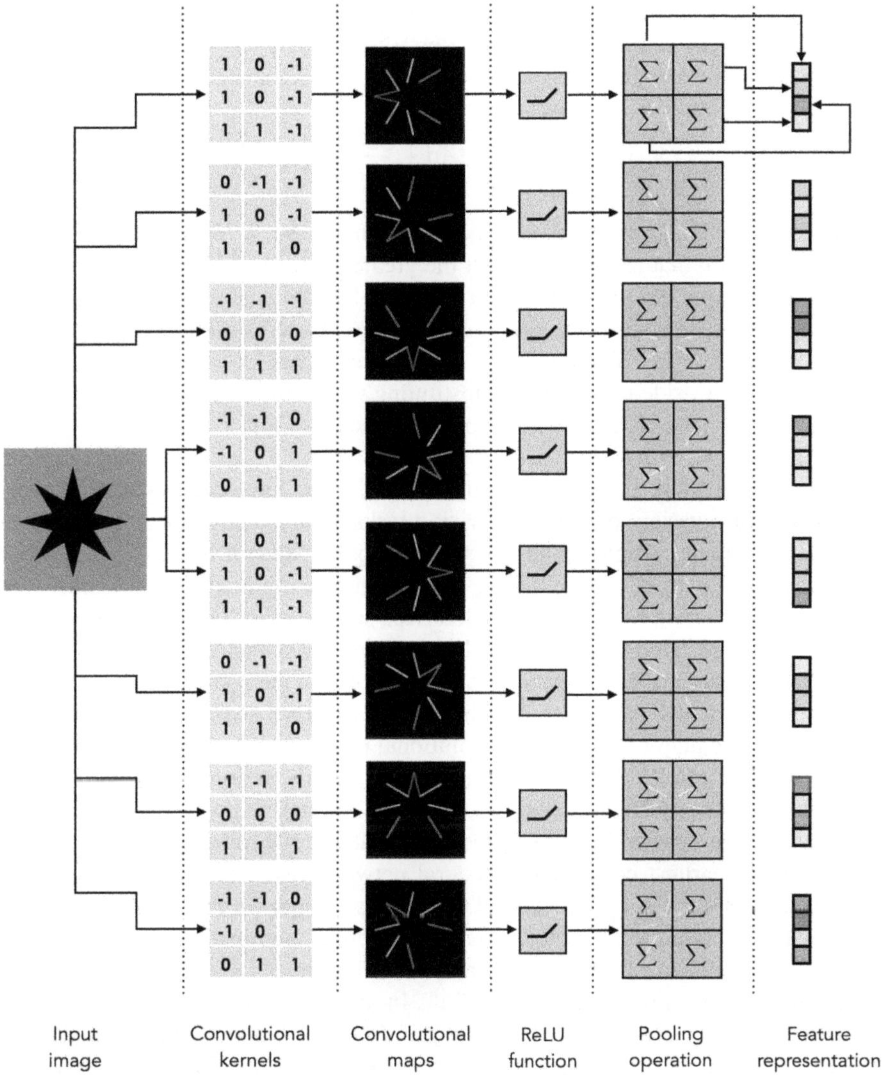

Fig. 7.15 Illustration of the edge-based feature extraction pipeline

In Fig. 7.15, we show the end-to-end edge-based feature extraction pipeline after the introduction of the pooling layer.

The feature extraction scheme shown in Fig. 7.15 has several adjustable hyper-parameters including:

- The number of convolution kernels, k
- The dimension of the convolutional kernels, $q \times q$
- The dimension of the pooling windows, $r \times r$
- The pooling stride, s

These hyperparameters are all discrete in nature and are usually tuned by trial and error. The choice of these hyperparameters directly impacts the total number of features in the final feature representation vector, which can be computed as

$$k\left(\left\lfloor \frac{N_1 - r}{s} \right\rfloor + 1\right)\left(\left\lfloor \frac{N_2 - r}{s} \right\rfloor + 1\right), \tag{7.20}$$

where the input image is assumed to be of dimension $N_1 \times N_2$, and $\lfloor \cdot \rfloor$ represents the floor function that returns as output the greatest integer less than or equal to its input. For example, the input image in Fig. 7.15 has dimensions $N_1 = N_2 = 512$. The feature extractor shown in the figure has $k = 8$ convolutional kernels of size 3×3 (hence, $q = 3$). The pooling windows are of size 256×256 each (hence, $r = 256$), with a stride of $s = 256$. Substituting these numbers into (7.20) gives 32 as the total number of features for the pipeline shown in Fig. 7.15.

In Fig. 7.15, we built a very basic pipeline for extracting edge-based features from an input image. More elaborate variations of this idea have been used effectively in practice for a variety of computer vision tasks [6, 7]. While these schemes are considerably more complex than the simple pipeline shown in Fig. 7.15, at their heart, they still extract features using fixed kernels similar to the ones shown in Fig. 7.12. In other words, the kernel matrices used in this breed of "engineered feature extractors" are predefined and do not change based on the input data.

A simple convolutional neural network (illustrated in the bottom row of Fig. 7.16) is different from the fixed-kernel architectures we have seen so far (top row of Fig. 7.16) in one major way: with convolutional neural networks, the kernels are no longer *fixed* but are instead *learned* (or tuned) using the training data. This means that unlike engineered feature extractors, convolutional neural networks have the capacity to learn optimal features from the data during the training process.

One of the earliest convolutional neural networks was the LeNet architecture, developed at Bell Labs by LeCun and colleagues [8] during the 1980s and 1990s. Designed for solving the computer vision problem of automatic digit recognition, the LeNet architecture takes as input a low-resolution (32×32 pixel) image of a handwritten digit, as illustrated in Fig. 7.17. In the first convolutional layer, $k_1 = 6$ kernels of size 5×5 are learned, resulting in 6 corresponding convolutional maps of size 28×28.[6] These maps were then passed through a sigmoid function[7] and subsequently pooled using a pooling stride of $s = 2$ to form 6 pooled maps of size 14×14. In the second convolutional layer, this process is repeated this time using $k_2 = 16$ convolutional kernels of size 5×5 (the pooling stride remains $s = 2$ as in the previous layer). The output of the second convolutional layer is then flattened into a column vector and fed into a fully connected multi-layer perceptron with

[6] In the original LeNet, convolutions were performed without padding the input. As a result, the output of the convolution was slightly smaller compared to the input.

[7] See Sect. "The Logistic Function" for a refresher. The sigmoid function was later replaced with ReLU in more modern convolutional neural network architectures.

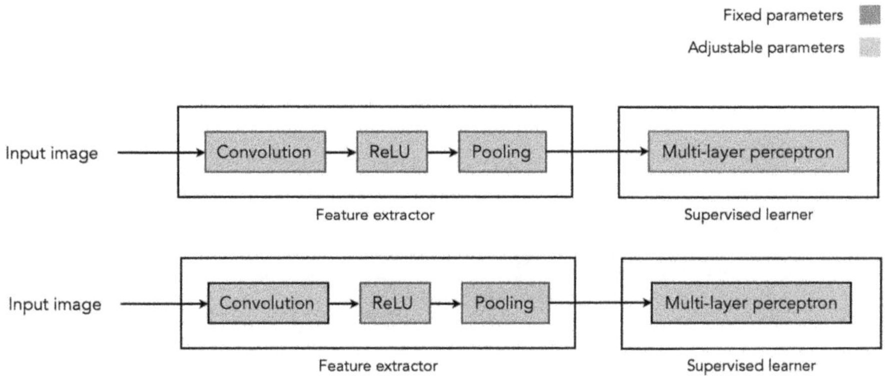

Fig. 7.16 Two high-level architectures for machine learning tasks involving image data. (Top row) A fixed feature extractor layer (consisting of fixed convolutional kernels, ReLU, and pooling modules) is inserted between the input image and the final multi-layer perceptron regressor/classifier. (Bottom row) In a convolutional neural network, the convolutional kernels in the feature extractor layer are tuned jointly with the multi-layer perceptron weights. The modules involving fixed and adjustable weights are colored gray and green, respectively

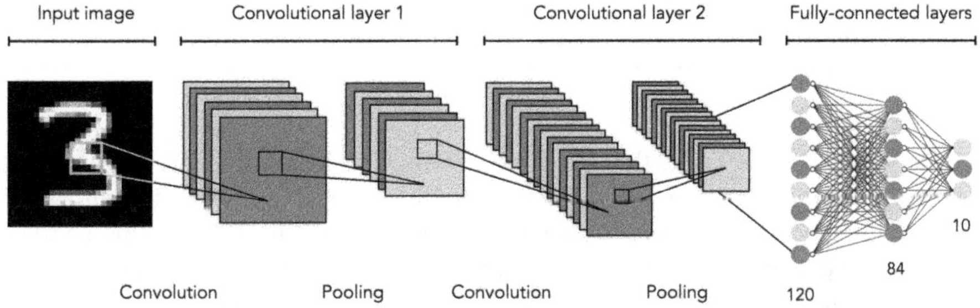

Fig. 7.17 An illustration of the LeNet [8] convolutional neural network

three layers. The first, second, and third layers consist of 120, 84, and 10 units, respectively.

In the top panel of Fig. 7.18, we show a more compact visual representation of the LeNet architecture, focusing on the number and size of convolutional kernels as well as the pooling window size and stride in each convolutional layer. The convolutional kernels and pooling windows are drawn exactly to size, and colored yellow and blue, respectively, while the fully connected layers are drawn as red circles. The number of convolutional kernels in each layer and the number of neuronal units in each fully connected layer are printed underneath them in brackets. The compact visual representation introduced here allows us to easily compare the classical LeNet with more modern convolutional neural network architectures such as the AlexNet [9] (middle panel of Fig. 7.18) and VGGNet [10] (bottom panel of Fig. 7.18).

Modern convolutional neural networks have tens of millions of tunable parameters distributed throughout both the convolutional and fully connected layers of

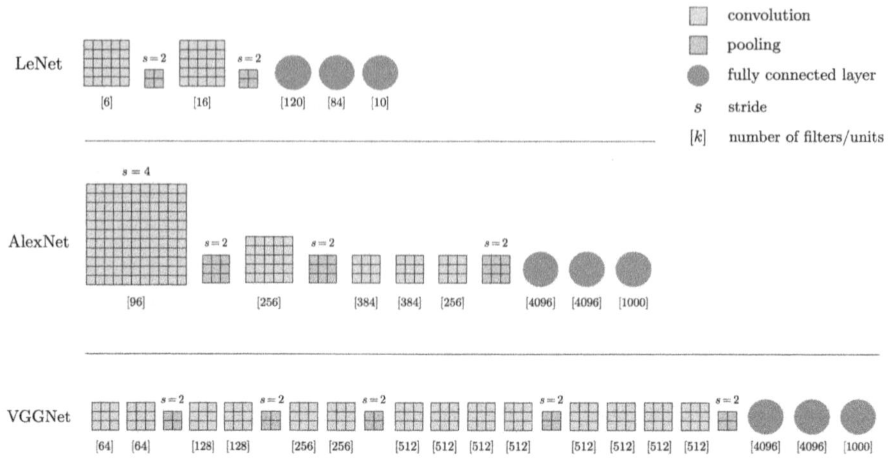

Fig. 7.18 The compact visual representations of three popular convolutional neural network architectures. (Top panel) The LeNet architecture has 2 convolutional layers and 3 fully connected layers. This model was originally trained on the MNIST dataset [11] consisting of 60,000 images of handwritten digits. (Middle panel) The AlexNet has 5 convolutional layers and 3 fully connected layers. This model was first trained on a subset of the ImageNet dataset [12] consisting of 1,200,000 natural images. (Bottom panel) The original VGGNet architecture consisted of 14 convolutional layers and 3 fully connected layers

the network. For example, the AlexNet (shown in the middle panel of Fig. 7.18) has roughly 60 million tunable weights, while this number is around 140 million in the case of the VGGNet (shown in the bottom panel of Fig. 7.18). In the absence of very large datasets (with hundreds of thousands or millions of data points), these architectures are extremely prone to overfitting. Additionally, training these deep architectures requires extensive computational resources and training time. For instance, the original AlexNet was trained on 2 GPU for 6 days, while the VGGNet was trained on 4 GPUs over a period of 2 weeks.

When the size of data is smaller than ideal and/or we have limited computational resources at our disposal to train a modern convolutional neural network from scratch, we can still leverage pre-trained models such as AlexNet or VGGNet by "transferring some of the knowledge" gained from these models to ours. This strategy is typically called *transfer learning*.

For instance, we can choose to re-use these pre-trained models by keeping all their weights untouched—except for the weights of the final fully connected layer that you can tune using our own (smaller) dataset. Depending on the size of our training data, we can take this idea one step further and also learn some of the weights in the convolutional layers, typically those belonging to the layers that are closer to the output. During the training phase of transfer learning, it is usually beneficial not to randomly re-initialize the weights we look to re-tune, but instead initialize them at their optimal values according to the pre-trained model (e.g., AlexNet or VGGNet).

Recurrence Relations

As we saw in Chap. 2, various types of medical data arise sequentially in an ordered fashion. These include time-series, text, and genome-sequencing data, to name a few. This kind of data is sometimes referred to as *dynamic* to contrast it with *static* data that is generated in no particular order. While we can continue to apply the standard machine learning tools discussed in the previous chapters to deal with dynamic data, the fact that it has this additional structure begs the question: can we leverage this structure to our advantage? This is very much akin to our discussion of convolutional neural networks earlier in the chapter where we injected the convolution operation into the neural network architecture in order to leverage the local spatial correlation that exists in imaging data. Here, and by analogy, we look at how to codify and leverage the sequential order that exists in dynamic data in order to design a new class of neural network architectures, called recurrent neural networks, tailored to handle such data. We begin this section by introducing fixed order dynamic systems as the most fundamental mathematical tool for modeling dynamic datasets.

As we discussed in detail in Sect. "The Convolution Operation", when analyzing a time-series dataset such as the one shown in Fig. 7.4, it is quite common to denoise it first. We saw (in the context of one-dimensional convolution) that one way to smooth out this type of data is via a moving (or sliding) average, where we take a small window and slide it along the time-series from start to finish. Taking the average inside of each sliding window tends to cancel out noisy values, resulting in a smoothed version of the original series that is easier to visualize and study.

Here, we follow the same steps laid out in Eqs. (7.2) through (7.6) using a slightly different notation that is commonly used in the study of recurrent neural networks. Denoting the original time-series by $x_1, x_2, \ldots, x_N$, the moving average—a time-series itself—can be expressed as

$$h_t = \begin{cases} x_t & t = 1, \ldots, L-1 \\ \frac{1}{L}\sum_{i=0}^{L-1} x_{t-i} & t = L, \ldots, N \end{cases}, \tag{7.21}$$

where the first $L - 1$ values of the moving average h are set to the values of the input time-series x itself. After these initial values, we create those that follow by averaging the preceding L elements of the input series. This simple moving average process is a popular example of dynamic systems with fixed order. The *dynamic systems* part of this phrase refers to the fact that the system h is defined in terms of recent values of the input sequence x. The *fixed order* part refers to just how many preceding elements of input x are used to calculate the values in h. In (7.21), this value was set to L for each value of h_t created (after the initial values).

The generic form of a dynamic system with fixed order is very similar to the moving average process expressed in (7.21); only it employs a general (and possibly nonlinear) function $f(\cdot)$ in place of the simple averaging function in order to combine a window of $L-1$ prior elements of an input sequence, as

$$h_t = \begin{cases} \gamma_t & t = 1, \ldots, L-1 \\ \\ f(x_t, \ldots, x_{t-L+1}) & t = L, \ldots, N \end{cases}. \tag{7.22}$$

Here, L is the *fixed order* of the dynamic system, and the first $L-1$ values $\gamma_1, \gamma_2, \ldots, \gamma_{L-1}$ are called the *initial conditions* of the system. These initial conditions are often dependent on the input sequence but, in general, can be set to any values. Fixed order dynamic systems are used in a variety of scientific and engineering disciplines. Convolutional operations, for instance, are prime examples of a dynamic system with fixed order and are frequently used to filter and adjust digital signals. A special case of a dynamic system with fixed order is when L is set to 1, implying that each element of the output sequence h_t is dependent only on the current input point x_t, that is, $h_t = f(x_t)$. These kinds of systems are called *memoryless* since the dynamic system is constructed without any knowledge of the past input values.

Another special class of fixed order dynamic systems are recurrence relations, where instead of constructing an output sequence based on a given input sequence, these systems define an input sequence in terms of itself, as

$$x_t = f(x_{t-1}, \ldots, x_{t-L}) \qquad t = L+1, \ldots, N. \tag{7.23}$$

In this case, we do not begin with an input sequence x and filter it to create an output sequence h. Instead, we *generate* the input itself by recursing on a set of formula of the form shown in (7.23). As such, these recurrence relations are sometimes referred to as *generative models*. Notice that with recurrence relations the initial conditions will still have to be set, which are simply the first $L-1$ entries of the input sequence.

Example 7.4 (Exponential Growth Modeling) The following simple recurrence relation of order $L = 1$

$$\begin{aligned} x_1 &= \gamma \\ x_t &= w_0 + w_1 x_{t-1} \end{aligned} \tag{7.24}$$

generates a sequence that exhibits exponential growth using the linear function $f(x) = w_0 + w_1 x$. Here, γ, w_0, and w_1 are all adjustable scalars.

In Fig. 7.19, we show two example sequences of length $N = 10$ generated using (7.24). In the first instance shown in the left panel of Fig. 7.19, we set the

(continued)

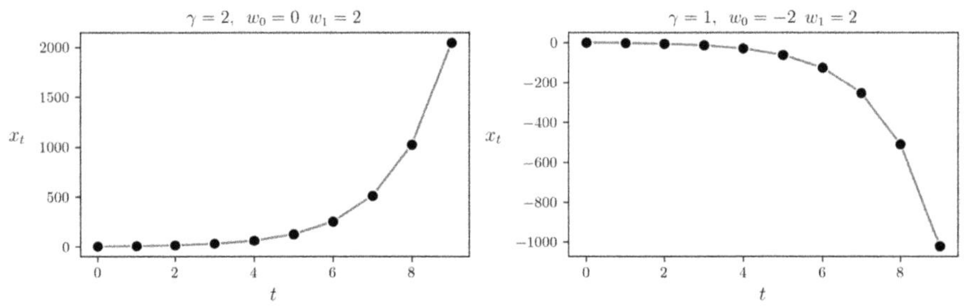

Fig. 7.19 Figure associated with Example 7.4. See text for details

Example 7.4 (continued)
initial condition and the linear function's weights as follows: $\gamma = 2$, $w_0 = 0$, and $w_1 = 2$. This results in an exponentially increasing sequence. In the right panel of the figure, we use another setting of the initial condition and the linear weights, i.e., $\gamma = 1$, $w_0 = -2$, and $w_1 = 2$, which leads to (this time) an exponentially decreasing sequence.

Supposing for the moment that $w_0 = 0$, we can *roll back* the recursion in (7.24) by replacing x_{t-1} with its recursive definition, i.e., $x_{t-1} = w_0 + w_1 x_{t-2} = w_1 x_{t-2}$, and write x_t as

$$x_t = w_1 \left(w_1 x_{t-2}\right) = w_1^2 x_{t-2}. \tag{7.25}$$

If we repeat this process, substituting in the recursive formula for x_{t-2}, then x_{t-3}, and so on, we can connect x_t all the way back to the initial condition, and write

$$x_t = w_1^t x_1 = w_1^t \gamma, \tag{7.26}$$

which shows how the sequence behaves exponentially depending on the value of w_1. If $w_0 \neq 0$, a similar exponential relationship can be derived by rolling back to the initial condition (see Exercise 7.6). As we saw previously in Sect. "The Logistic Function", this sort of dynamic system arises in Malthusian modeling of population growth.

Example 7.5 (Auto-Regressive Modeling) One extension of the exponential growth model in Example 7.4 is the so-called *auto-regressive* system, wherein the recursive update formula consists of a linear combination of L prior

(continued)

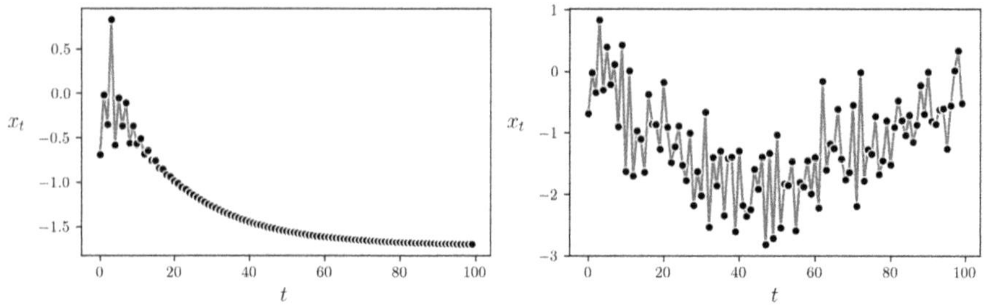

Fig. 7.20 Figure associated with Example 7.5. See text for details

Example 7.5 (continued)
elements in the input sequence (with the addition of some small amount of noise). An auto-regressive system of order L takes the general form of

$$\begin{aligned} x_1 &= \gamma_1, \\ x_2 &= \gamma_2, \\ &\vdots \\ x_L &= \gamma_L, \\ x_t &= w_0 + \left(\sum_{i=1}^{L} w_i \, x_{t-i} \right) + \epsilon_t, \quad \text{if } t > L, \end{aligned} \tag{7.27}$$

where ϵ_t denotes the small amount of added noise introduced at each step. In Fig. 7.20, we show two sequences generated via the auto-regressive system in (7.27). In both cases, $L = 4$, and we have used the same initial conditions and linear function weights. The only difference between the two sequences is the value of ϵ_t in each case. In the left panel, no noise was added, i.e., $\epsilon_t = 0$, while a small random (Gaussian) noise was added to the sequence shown in the right panel.

Another classic example of an auto-regressive model is the Fibonacci sequence, defined recursively as

$$\begin{aligned} x_1 &= 0 \\ x_2 &= 1 \\ x_t &= x_{t-1} + x_{t-2} \quad \text{if } t > 2, \end{aligned} \tag{7.28}$$

which is a special case of (7.27) with $L = 2$, $\gamma_1 = 0$, $\gamma_2 = 1$, $w_0 = 0$, $w_1 = 1$, and $w_2 = 1$, and $\epsilon_t = 0$.

Example 7.6 (Chaotic Modeling) Here, we illustrate several examples of the sort of recurrence relations that can be generated via the following dynamic system of order $L = 1$

$$\begin{aligned} x_1 &= \gamma \\ x_t &= w x_{t-1} \left(1 - x_{t-1}\right), \end{aligned} \tag{7.29}$$

where the recursive update function is no longer linear, but quadratic. Take a moment to revisit Sect. "The Logistic Function", and notice the similarity between the dynamic system in (7.29) and the differential equation in (5.6). In fact, using the right settings of γ and w, we can generate the familiar s-shaped logistic curve, as illustrated in Fig. 7.21,

This dynamic system is often *chaotic*, meaning that slight adjustments to the initial condition γ and weight w can produce drastically different results. For instance, in Fig. 7.22, we show two sequences with the same initial condition $\gamma = 10^{-4}$ but different weight values: in the left panel $w = 3$, while in the right panel $w = 4$. As can be seen from comparing the two panels, a relatively small change in w can turn a nicely converging sequence (left) into a chaotic pseudo-random one (right).

The Examples 7.4–7.6 showcase a universal property of recurrence relations: their behavior is heavily influenced by their initial conditions. This fact becomes clear if we "roll back" the system starting at x_t. Suppose for simplicity that $L = 1$ and that $x_t = f(x_{t-1})$ for some function f. Using this recursive definition, we can directly connect x_t to the initial condition x_1 via

$$x_t = f\left(f\left(\cdots f\left(x_1\right)\right)\cdots\right) = f^{(t-1)}\left(x_1\right), \tag{7.30}$$

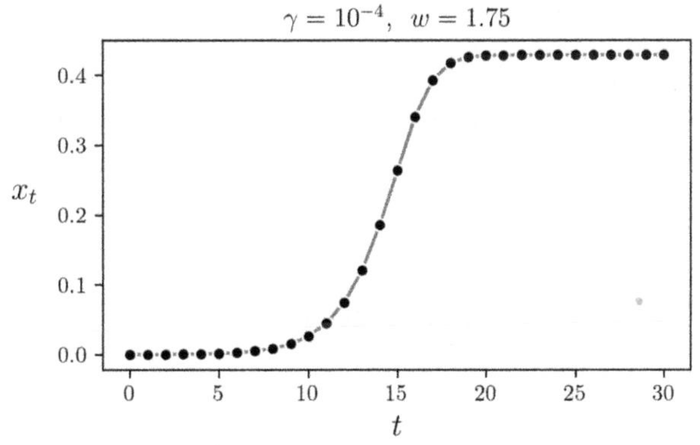

Fig. 7.21 An illustration of the logistic sequence generated via (7.29) using $\gamma = 10^{-4}$ and $w = 1.75$

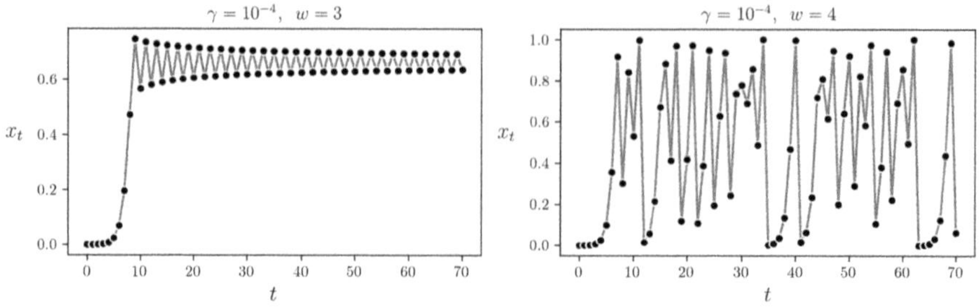

Fig. 7.22 Figure associated with Example 7.6. See text for details

where we have composed f with itself t times. This confirms that every point in a sequence generated by a recurrence relation of order $L = 1$ is completely determined by its initial condition. The same is true in general for recurrence relations with order $L > 1$.

It is important to note that from the very definition of a recurrence relation with order L

$$x_t = f(x_{t-1}, \ldots, x_{t-L}), \tag{7.31}$$

we can see that each x_t is dependent on *only* the value of x_{t-1} through x_{t-L}, and no point coming before x_{t-L}. Therefore, the range of values used to build each subsequent point is—by definition—limited by the order of the system. Such systems with "limited memory" have two major disadvantages. First, it is often not easy to select a proper value for L. If set too small, the system may lack enough memory to model a recursive phenomenon. On the other hand, large values of L can result in needlessly complex models that are difficult to optimize and wield. Second—and more importantly—many modalities of dynamic data (e.g., text) can have variable length. Take patient notes for example. If you were to use patient notes to predict the health status of admitted patients in a hospital (i.e., a binary label that can be positive or negative), how would you choose a fixed value for L knowing that some patient notes can be only a few words long, while others can be quite lengthy, sometimes exceeding a few pages? Because a fixed order dynamic system is limited by its order and cannot use any information from earlier in a sequence, this problem can arise regardless of the order L that we choose. In the next section, we introduce variable order dynamic systems to remedy this problem.

Recurrent Neural Networks

Previously, we discussed the *moving average* as a prototypical example of a dynamic system with fixed order. In this section, we introduce the *exponential average* as a prototype for dynamic systems with variable order. In the case of the latter averaging scheme, instead of taking a sliding window and averaging the input series inside of it, we compute the average of the entire input sequence in an online fashion, adding the contribution of each input one element at a time. Before discussing how the exponential average is computed, it is helpful to first define a *running average* for the input sequence $x_1, x_2, \ldots, x_N$, as follows:

$$\begin{aligned}
h_1 &= x_1 \\
h_2 &= \frac{x_1 + x_2}{2} \\
h_3 &= \frac{x_1 + x_2 + x_3}{3} \\
&\vdots \\
h_N &= \frac{x_1 + x_2 + \cdots + x_N}{N}.
\end{aligned} \tag{7.32}$$

Here, each point h_t in the running average sequence is the arithmetic average of all points in the input sequence indexed from 1 to t. In other words, the running average sequence h_t *summarizes* the input sequence up to (and including) x_t via a simple summary statistic: their sample mean.

Notice that the running average in (7.32) is a dynamic system that can be written recursively as

$$h_t = \left(\frac{t-1}{t}\right) h_{t-1} + \frac{1}{t} x_t \tag{7.33}$$

for all $t = 1, 2, \ldots, N$. Once you have taken a moment to verify that (7.32) and (7.33) are indeed equivalent, also notice that h_t does not have a fixed order as h_1 depends only on one input point, h_2 depends on two input points, h_3 depends on three input points, and so forth. If h_t was a fixed order system, then its value would depend on the same number of input points at all steps.

While (7.32) and (7.33) are two equivalent representations of the same dynamic system, the latter is far more efficient from a computational perspective. To see why this is the case, let us compute the entire running average sequence $h_1, h_2, \ldots, h_N$ using both representations, counting the number of mathematical operations (addition, multiplication, division, etc.) that must be performed along the way. Using (7.32), we need no additions or divisions to compute h_1, 1 addition and 1 division to compute h_2, 2 additions and 1 division to compute h_3, and so on, totaling

$$0 + 1 + 2 + \cdots + (N-1) = \frac{1}{2}(N-1)N \tag{7.34}$$

additions and $N-1$ divisions overall. Note that the number of additions is *quadratic* in N, making it prohibitively large as N grows larger. On the other hand, using the definition in (7.33), we need to perform a constant number of operations (one addition, one multiplication, one division[8]) to compute the running average at each step, giving a total of $3N$ operations overall, which is linear in N and thus scales much more gracefully with the size of the input sequence.

Moreover, the recursive representation in (7.33) has a memory advantage over the *unfolded* or *unrolled* representation in (7.32). With the latter, when computing the running average h_t, we need access to explicit values of every value up to and including x_t (i.e., x_1 through x_t), whereas with the former we only need to access two values: x_t and h_{t-1}.

The *exponential average* is a simple generalization of the running average in (7.33) wherein h_{t-1} and x_t are linearly combined using a different set of weights or coefficients. More specifically, instead of multiplying h_{t-1} and x_t by $\frac{t-1}{t}$ and $\frac{1}{t}$, and summing the result, we multiply them by α and $1 - \alpha$, respectively, where α is a scalar parameter that is kept fixed at each step. Expressed algebraically, we have

$$h_t = \alpha\, h_{t-1} + (1 - \alpha)\, x_t. \tag{7.35}$$

This slightly adjusted version of the running average is called an exponential average because if we roll (7.35) back to its initial condition—as we did in (7.26)—the following exponentially weighted average emerges (see Exercise 7.7)

$$h_t = \alpha^t\, x_1 + \alpha^{t-1}\, (1 - \alpha)\, x_2 + \cdots + \alpha\, (1 - \alpha)\, x_{t-1} + (1 - \alpha)\, x_t. \tag{7.36}$$

The generic form of a dynamic system with variable order is very similar to the exponential average shown in (7.36) and can be written as

$$\begin{aligned} h_1 &= \gamma\,(x_1) \\ h_t &= f\,(h_{t-1}, x_t) \qquad t > 1, \end{aligned} \tag{7.37}$$

where $\gamma\,(\cdot)$ and $f\,(\cdot)$ can be any mathematical function. While there are many variations on this generic theme, all dynamic systems with variable order share the two universal properties: first, h_t is defined recursively in itself, and second, it provides a summary of all preceding input values x_1 through x_t and as such is sometimes referred to as the *state* variable in the context of variable order dynamic systems. We can see why this is the case if we roll back h_t in (7.37) all the way to h_1, via

$$h_t = f\,(f\,(f\,(\cdots f\,(\gamma\,(x_1)\,, x_2)\,, x_3) \cdots\,, x_{t-1})\,, x_t)\,, \tag{7.38}$$

[8] This can be seen more clearly if we write (7.33) as

$$h_t = \frac{(t - 1)\, h_{t-1} + x_t}{t}.$$

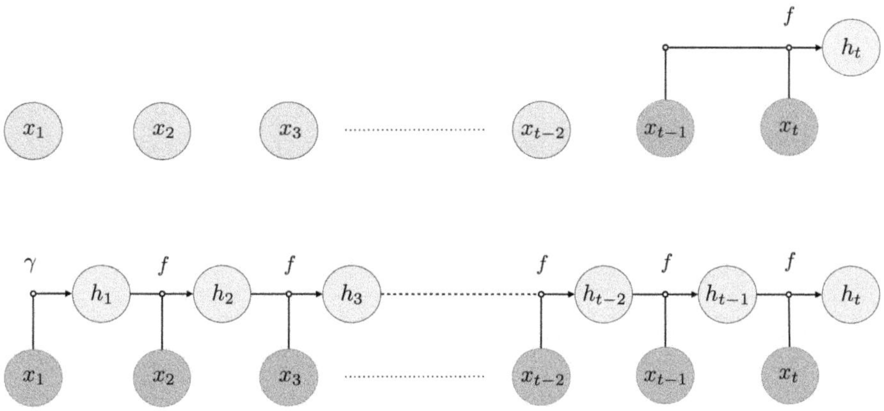

Fig. 7.23 Graphical model representations of dynamic systems with fixed and variable order. (Top panel) The memory of a fixed order dynamic system is limited to the order of the system L, meaning that the system is only aware of the most recent L elements of the input sequence. Here $L = 2$, and the input points that play a role in the value of h_t are colored in red. (Bottom panel) The memory of a variable order dynamic system is *complete* in the sense that every preceding input plays a role in determining the value of the output at time or step t

which exposes the fact that h_t is dependent on all prior values of the input sequence x_1 through x_t. In other words, at each step, h_t provides a summary of the input up to that point in the sequence, and therefore, it has a "full memory" of all input preceding it. This is in direct contrast to the fixed order dynamic system described in the previous section where every value was dependent on only a fixed and limited number of inputs preceding it. This comparison is illustrated in Fig. 7.23.

The variable order dynamic system shown in the bottom panel of Fig. 7.23 provides a blueprint for building a recurrent neural network, a prototypical example of which is illustrated in Fig. 7.24. Here, in addition to the input sequence (in red) and the state sequence (in yellow), we have an output sequence (in blue) sitting atop the state layer. Unlike the representation in the bottom panel of Fig. 7.23 wherein the function f remains the same throughout the system, in recurrent neural networks, f can change from state to state. In practice, however, f_i's tend to have the same functional form but use different parameters. For example,

$$\begin{aligned} f_1(h_1, x_2) &= \tanh\left(v_1 h_1 + w_1 x_2\right) \\ f_2(h_2, x_3) &= \tanh\left(v_2 h_2 + w_2 x_3\right) \\ &\vdots \\ f_{t-1}(h_{t-1}, x_t) &= \tanh\left(v_{t-1} h_{t-1} + w_{t-1} x_t\right) \end{aligned} \tag{7.39}$$

is a common choice for the functions f_1 through f_{t-1} with v_i's and w_i's being tunable parameters. The same is true for the functions g_1 through g_t that predict the

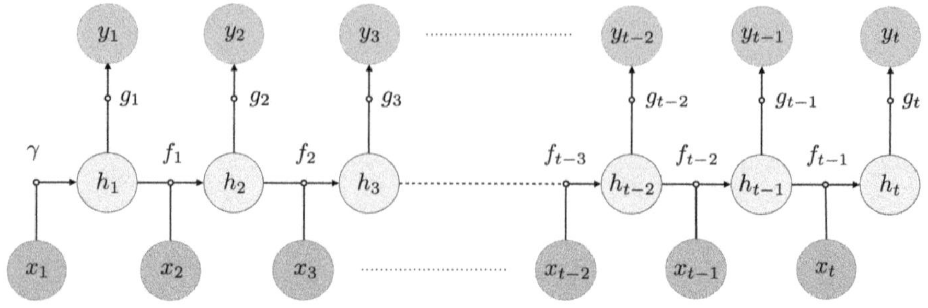

Fig. 7.24 A prototypical recurrent neural network

outputs y_1 through y_t from the states h_1 through h_t. As with any other machine learning and deep learning model we have encountered so far, all the function parameters must be learned during training.

Finally, it should be noted that sometimes—and depending on the application—the output of a recurrent neural network is not a sequence but a single variable. For instance, in classification tasks involving dynamic or sequential data, we can remove all the output points y_1 through y_{t-1} from the architecture in Fig. 7.24, keeping only y_t that will contain the predicted classification label.

Problems

7.1 Image Denoising

In Example 7.1, we used one-dimensional convolution to denoise the Covid-19 time-series data plotted in Fig. 7.4. In this exercise, you will apply two-dimensional convolution to perform denoising on a two-dimensional piece of data: the chest X-ray shown in Fig. 7.25. The left panel of the figure shows the original (i.e., clean) image along with two noisy versions of it in the middle and right panels, corrupted by a moderate and high level of noise, respectively. Specifically, you will convolve each noisy image with one uniform convolutional kernel

$$w = \frac{1}{(2\ell+1)^2} \begin{bmatrix} 1 & 1 & \cdots & 1 \\ 1 & 1 & \cdots & 1 \\ \vdots & \vdots & \ddots & \vdots \\ 1 & 1 & \cdots & 1 \end{bmatrix}_{(2\ell+1)\times(2\ell+1)}$$

and one non-uniform convolutional kernel

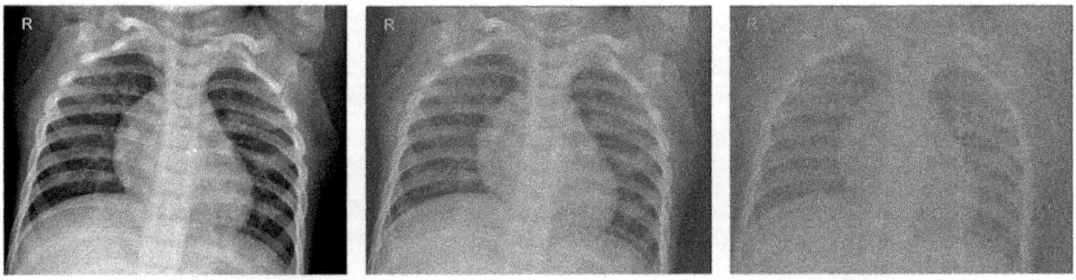

Fig. 7.25 Figure associated with Exercise 7.1. The three images shown here can be downloaded from the chapter's supplements

$$w = \frac{1}{L}\begin{bmatrix} 1 & 2 & \cdots & \ell & \ell+1 & \ell & \cdots & 2 & 1 \\ 2 & 3 & \cdots & \ell+1 & \ell+2 & \ell+1 & \cdots & 3 & 2 \\ \vdots & \vdots & \ddots & \vdots & \vdots & \vdots & \ddots & \vdots & \vdots \\ \ell & \ell+1 & \cdots & 2\ell-1 & 2\ell & 2\ell-1 & \cdots & \ell+1 & \ell \\ \ell+1 & \ell+2 & \cdots & 2\ell & 2\ell+1 & 2\ell & \cdots & \ell+2 & \ell+1 \\ \ell & \ell+1 & \cdots & 2\ell-1 & 2\ell & 2\ell-1 & \cdots & \ell+1 & \ell \\ \vdots & \vdots & \ddots & \vdots & \vdots & \vdots & \ddots & \vdots & \vdots \\ 2 & 3 & \cdots & \ell+1 & \ell+2 & \ell+1 & \cdots & 3 & 2 \\ 1 & 2 & \cdots & \ell & \ell+1 & \ell & \cdots & 2 & 1 \end{bmatrix},$$

where $L = (2\ell+1)(2\ell^2+2\ell+1)$, for a range of different values of ℓ in each case:

(a) Which kernel type (uniform or non-uniform) provided the best result overall?
(b) Which kernel size ℓ provided the best result on the moderately noisy image?
(c) Which kernel size ℓ provided the best result on the highly noisy image?
(d) Are your answers to parts (b) and (c) the same? If not, explain why.

7.2 Edge Detection Using Convolution

Find the output image resulting from the convolution of the image/matrix shown in Fig. 7.26 with each of the following kernels:

(a) $w_1 = \begin{bmatrix} +1 & 0 & -1 \\ +1 & 0 & -1 \\ +1 & 0 & -1 \end{bmatrix}.$

(b) $w_2 = \begin{bmatrix} +1 & +1 & +1 \\ 0 & 0 & 0 \\ -1 & -1 & -1 \end{bmatrix}.$

(c) $w_3 = \begin{bmatrix} +1 & +1 & 0 \\ +1 & 0 & -1 \\ 0 & -1 & -1 \end{bmatrix}.$

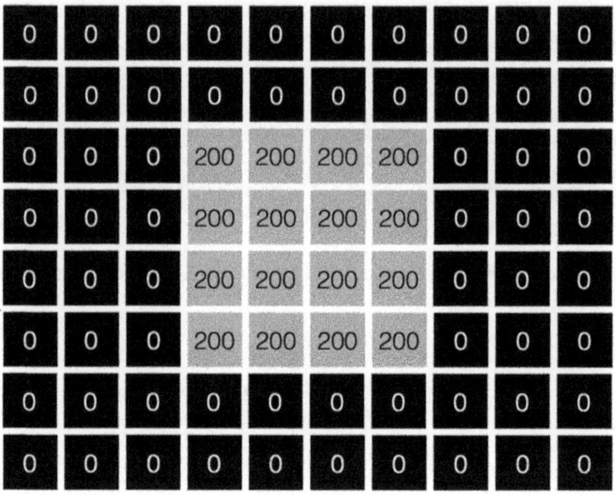

Fig. 7.26 Figure associated with Exercise 7.3

7.3 Circular Imperfection

Can you explain why the edge-based feature representation of the circle shown in the middle panel of Fig. 7.13 is not perfectly uniform (meaning that some edge directions contain more "energy" than the others)?

7.4 Computing the Number of Parameters in a Convolutional Neural Network

Compute the total number of adjustable parameters for the classic convolutional neural networks depicted in Fig. 7.18, using the formula in (7.20) along with the descriptions of LeNet in [8], AlexNet in [9], and VGGNet in [10].

7.5 Identifying Recurrence in a Numerical Sequence

We saw in the chapter that the so-called Fibonacci sequence

$$0, 1, 1, 2, 3, 5, 8, 13, 21, 34, 55, \ldots$$

is defined recursively via

$$\begin{aligned} x_1 &= 0 \\ x_2 &= 1 \\ x_t &= x_{t-1} + x_{t-2} \quad \text{if } t > 2. \end{aligned}$$

For each of the following sequences, can you define a similar recursive formula that generates the entire sequence starting from some initial condition? If not, why?

(a) $1, 1, 2, 4, 7, 13, 24, 44, 81, \ldots$
(b) $1, 2, 4, 8, 16, 32, 64, 128, \ldots$
(c) $1, 2, 6, 24, 120, 720, 5040, \ldots$
(d) $2, 3, 5, 7, 11, 13, 17, 19, 23, 29, \ldots$

7.6 Rolling Back Exponential Growth

In Example 7.4, we rolled back the recursion in (7.24) assuming $w_0 = 0$ and connected x_t to the system's initial condition as shown in (7.26). Follow a similar set of steps to roll back the recursion in general, i.e., without assuming $w_0 = 0$.

7.7 Rolling Back Exponential Average

Verify that rolling (7.35) back to its initial condition yields the exponentially weighted average shown in (7.36).

7.8 A Dynamic System for Monitoring Blood Glucose Level

Diabetic patients monitor their blood glucose level regularly to ensure it always falls within a desired range. Denoting by x_t the blood glucose level of a patient at time t, define a variable order dynamic system h_t for the historical maximum of the input sequence $x_1, x_2, x_3, \ldots, x_t$ using (7.37). In other words, define the functions $\gamma(\cdot)$ and $f(\cdot)$ such that at each step h_t represents the patient's highest recorded blood glucose level. Repeat the same for the historical minimum, i.e., the lowest recorded blood glucose level.

References

1. The New York Times. Coronavirus (Covid-19) Data in the United States. Accessed July 2022. https://github.com/nytimes/covid-19-data
2. Keshavamurthy J. Case study: bisphosphonate induced femur fractures. Accessed Aug 2022. https://doi.org/10.53347/rID-45453
3. Barlow H. Redundancy reduction revisited. Netw Comput Neural Syst. 2001;12(3):241–53
4. Marčelja S. Mathematical description of the responses of simple cortical cells. JOSA. 1980;70(11):1297–300
5. Jones JP, Palmer LA. An evaluation of the two-dimensional Gabor filter model of simple receptive fields in cat striate cortex. J Neurophysiol. 1987;58(6):1233–58.
6. Dalal N, Triggs B. Histograms of oriented gradients for human detection. Proc IEEE Comput Soc Conf Comput Vis Pattern Recognit. 2005;1:886–93
7. Lowe DG. Distinctive image features from scale-invariant keypoints. Int J Comput Vis. 2004;60(2):91–110
8. LeCun Y, Boser B, Denker JS, et al. Backpropagation applied to handwritten zip code recognition. Neural Comput. 1989;4(1):541–51
9. Krizhevsky A, Sutskever I, Hinton GE. ImageNet classification with deep convolutional neural networks. In: Proceedings of the 25th international conference on neural information processing systems. Vol. 1. NIPS'12. Red Hook: Curran Associates Inc.; 2012. p. 10971105
10. Simonyan K, Zisserman A. Very deep convolutional networks for large-scale image recognition. In: 3rd international conference on learning representations, ICLR 2015, San Diego, May 7–9, 2015. Conference Track Proceedings; 2015. Available from: http://arxiv.org/abs/1409.1556
11. Deng L. The MNIST database of handwritten digit images for machine learning research. IEEE Signal Proces Magaz. 2012;29(6):141–2
12. Deng J, Dong W, Socher R, Li LJ, Li K, Fei-Fei L. ImageNet: a large-scale hierarchical image database. In: 2009 IEEE conference on computer vision and pattern recognition. Piscataway: IEEE; 2009. p. 248–55

Chapter 8
Reinforcement Learning

Reinforcement learning is a general machine learning framework that is fundamentally different from the supervised learning frameworks discussed in the previous chapters. When trained properly, reinforcement learning allows computational agents to act intelligently in a complex (and often dynamic) environment in order to achieve a narrowly defined goal. Among the applications of this framework are game-playing AI (e.g., AlphaGo, Chess, and Atari/Nintendo games) as well as various challenging problems in robotics and automatic control. In medicine, reinforcement learning has been successfully applied to robotic-assisted surgery as well as to devising personalized treatment strategies for patients.

The sheer number of complex ideas involved in reinforcement learning makes it more challenging to grasp than the previously discussed supervised learning frameworks. That is why in this chapter, we introduce reinforcement learning by pulling apart the entire process and by introducing each concept as needed. By focusing our attention on just one piece of the system at a time, we can gain a fuller understanding of how each component works, and why it is needed. Moreover, by doing so, we also gain some extremely important intuition about how the individual components of reinforcement learning define the strengths and limitations of the process in general.

Reinforcement Learning Applications

We begin our discussion of the reinforcement learning framework by describing—at a high level—some of its common applications in several areas both within and outside medicine. These example applications represent the kind of tasks that can be performed using the reinforcement learning approach. We will return to these examples repeatedly throughout this chapter as we develop reinforcement learning concepts.

R. Borhani et al., *Fundamentals of Machine Learning and Deep Learning in Medicine*, https://doi.org/10.1007/978-3-031-19502-0_8

Path-Finding AI

Path-finding problems are commonly encountered in robotics applications as well as video games and mapping services. For many robots (e.g., a cleaning bot), path-finding is essential for efficient operation. In a video game, the enemy AI uses path-finding to reach human players in a level as quickly as possible. With a digital mapping service, path-finding is used to efficiently route you from point A to point B.

In this chapter, we will study a toy version of the path-finding problem, called Gridworld, wherein the robot (agent) must learn how to navigate a grid-like map efficiently in order to reach a target destination (goal) on the map. The left panel of Fig. 8.1 shows a simple example of Gridworld: a small maze. The black circle denotes the robot/agent, and the green square represents the desired destination. In the Gridworld environment, the robot can move one unit left, right, up, or down at a time, to any "safe" square (colored white). While the robot is also allowed to pass through the "hazard" squares (colored red), it would be heavily penalized for doing so, as these squares simulate hazardous locations (such as a slippery or obstructed part of the floor). Starting at any given location, the agent in Gridworld must learn the shortest path to the green square while avoiding hazards along the way.

It is important to note that in Gridworld the agent cannot "see" the entire map, the way it is depicted in the left panel of Fig. 8.1. From the agent's perspective, the world looks like the one shown in the figure's right panel where the robot can only see those parts of the map it is allowed to move into.

Gridworlds come in a variety of shapes and sizes. The left panel of Fig. 8.2 shows a small Gridworld where the hazards are arranged in a certain way to form a narrow passage separating one half of the grid from another. If the robot starts on the "wrong" side of the grid (as shown in the figure), then it must cross a narrow bridge to reach the green target. Another Gridworld example is depicted in the right

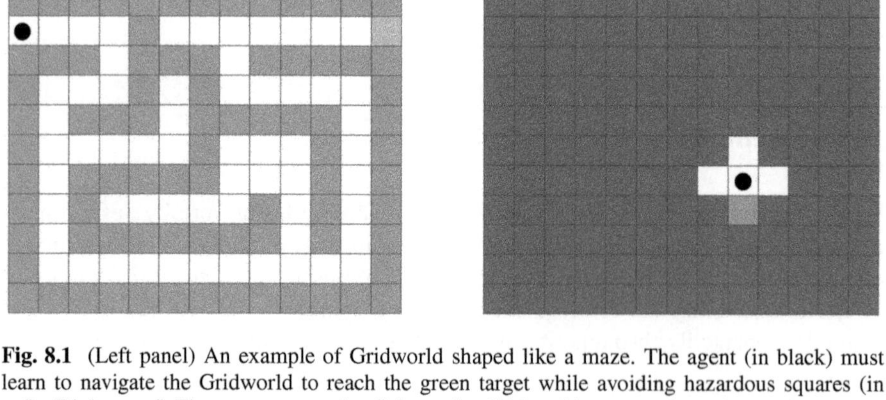

Fig. 8.1 (Left panel) An example of Gridworld shaped like a maze. The agent (in black) must learn to navigate the Gridworld to reach the green target while avoiding hazardous squares (in red). (Right panel) The agent cannot "see" the entire Gridworld at once. At each turn, it can only see neighboring squares to its current location

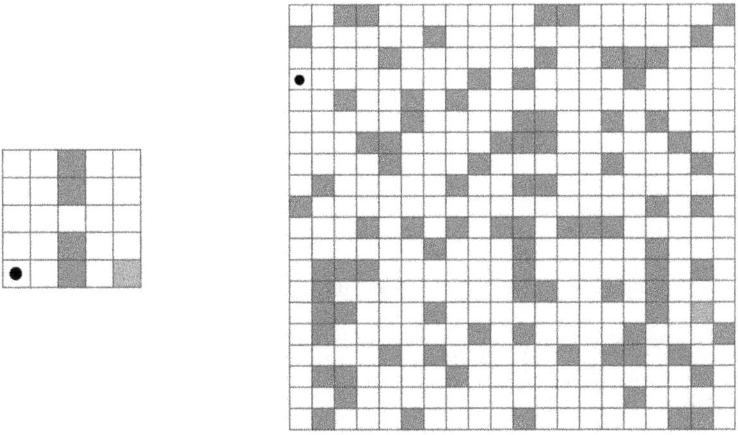

Fig. 8.2 (Left panel) A small 5 × 5 Gridworld where the hazard squares are organized in a particular way to divide the world into two halves, leaving only a narrow passage for the agent on the left to reach the target on the right. (Right panel) A larger 20 × 20 Gridworld with randomly placed hazards

panel of Fig. 8.2 where the world is considerably larger compared to the previous examples. Moreover, the hazards in this case are placed randomly and—as a result—do not seem to follow any specific pattern. Here, too, the robot must learn to navigate a hazard-free path to reach the green target efficiently.

Automatic Control

Many automatic control problems involve teaching an agent how to control a particular mechanical, electrical, or aerodynamic system. One classic example in this area is to teach an agent how to balance a pole on a moving cart, sometimes referred to as the cart–pole or inverted pendulum problem. As illustrated in the left panel of Fig. 8.3, the pole is free to rotate about an axis on the cart, with the cart on a track so that it may be moved left and right, affecting the location of the pole. The pole feels the force of the Earth's gravity and, if unbalanced, will fall to the ground.

Autopilot systems are another technology that can make use of reinforcement learning. A classic problem in this area is the so-called lunar lander, where the objective is to train a reinforcement learning agent that can correctly land a spacecraft in a certain landing zone between two red flags, as illustrated in the right panel of Fig. 8.3.

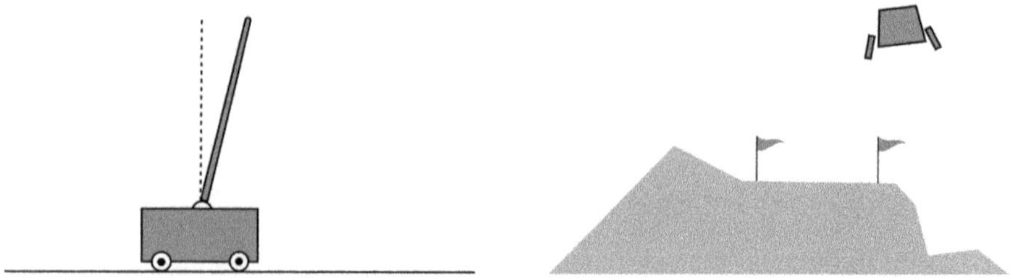

Fig. 8.3 An illustration of the cart–pole (left) and the lunar lander problem (right)

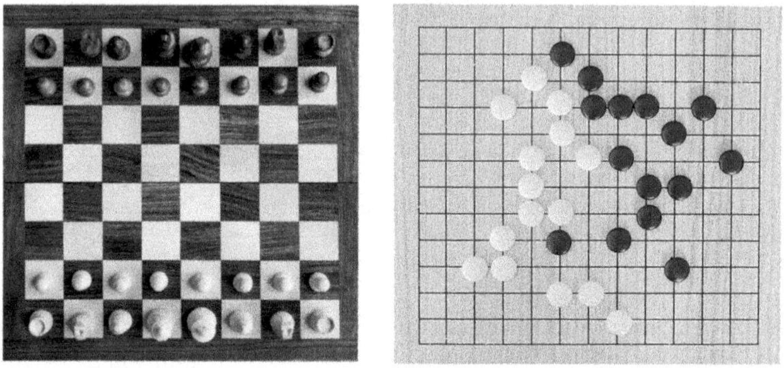

Fig. 8.4 Reinforcement learning can be used to train AI agents to play board games such as Chess (left panel) and Go (right panel)

Game-Playing AI

Another common application of reinforcement learning is to train AI agents to win certain video and board games. In the game of Chess (the left panel of Fig. 8.4) for instance, the objective is to train an agent that can consistently checkmate its opponent according to the rules of the game. In 2016, a reinforcement learning agent trained to play the game of Go (the right panel of Fig. 8.4) beat the strongest player in the world 4–1 in a five-game series of matches.

Autonomous Robotic Surgery

Autonomous robotic surgery is one of application areas of reinforcement learning in medicine where an agent is trained to perform certain surgical procedures with no human involvement. Figure 8.5 shows four snapshots taken during a laparoscopic surgery procedure performed by a pair of robotic arms. This procedure, known as *pattern-cutting*, involves cutting a circular pattern on a tissue phantom using a surgical cutter (the arm coming into the frame from the right) and a tissue gripper

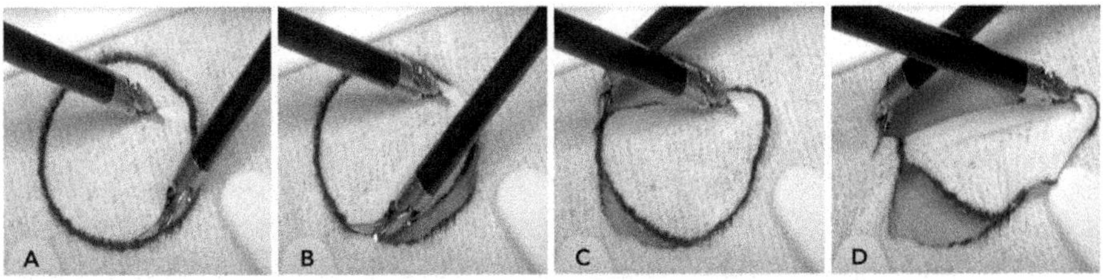

Fig. 8.5 The process of pattern-cutting performed by a pair of robotic arms trained using reinforcement learning. This figure was reproduced from [1]

(the arm coming into the frame from the left). The function of the gripper arm is to facilitate the procedure by grasping the soft tissue and applying forces of varying magnitude and direction to it as the other arm cuts through the tissue.

Automated Planning of Radiation Treatment

Radiation therapy is a common form of cancer treatment in which malignant tissues are irradiated using ionizing beams that are capable of destroying the DNA structure of cancerous cells. As illustrated in Fig. 8.6, accurate determination of the optimal dosage and angle of irradiation is crucial in the overall success of radiation therapy. If the impact zone of irradiation does not fully encircle the tumor and/or the dosage is too low or high, the therapy will not achieve its intended goal. It is important to note that any normal cell that is exposed to ionizing beams will also be damaged indiscriminately. Therefore, the objective of radiation therapy is to deliver a high enough dose to the tumor while minimizing radiation exposure to the surrounding healthy tissues.

Radiotherapy is typically administered over a period of time in multiple sessions in order to allow for normal cells to repair the damage caused by radiation. Traditionally, the same amount of radiation dose would be allocated to every session. This uniform dose distribution, however, is sub-optimal because tumors change dynamically over time. A dose that was appropriate for the first session may not be as effective in the second session. For instance, if the tumor does not respond favorably to the first dose, a higher dose may be warranted. On the other hand, the second dose may need to be lowered for a tumor that shrank significantly following the initial dose so as to minimize collateral damage to the surrounding normal cells. These inherent action–response dynamics at play here make reinforcement learning an ideal modeling approach for radiation therapy.

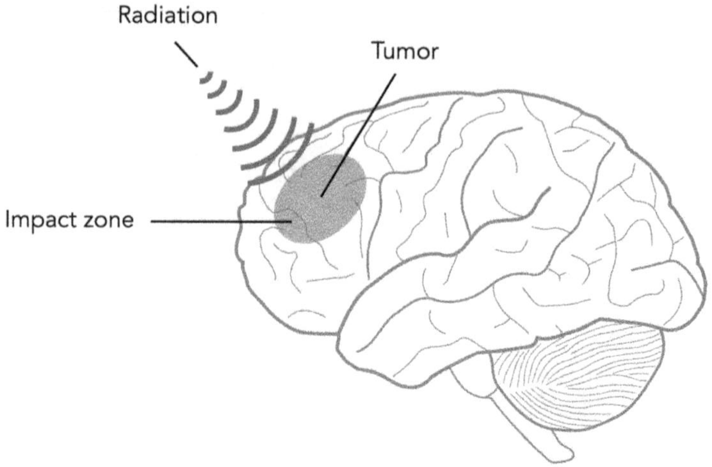

Fig. 8.6 The angle and dosage of radiation are important parameters in radiation therapy as they determine the impact zone of the ionizing beams as well as the level of energy delivered to the cells within that zone

Fundamental Concepts

The applications discussed in Sect. "Reinforcement Learning Applications", while seemingly quite different, share a common element: they all have narrowly defined goals that the reinforcement learning agent is trained to accomplish. With the autopilot system on an airplane for instance, the goal is to keep the plane flying safely toward a predefined destination. To achieve this goal, one could attempt to collect and code up a list of "if-then" type rules to solve this problem. However, the sheer amount of sensory data that must be factored in when compiling the list (plane's velocity, altitude, ambient air pressure, stress on various parts of the plane, etc.) would extremely complicate the process. Additionally, there are a myriad of environmental factors to deal with (e.g., air density, wind velocity, and currents) that can vary wildly from flight to flight.

The reinforcement learning approach ditches the notion of producing a long list of engineered conditionals to solve such a problem and instead trains a computational agent to accomplish the desired goal. To do this, the agent must have the ability to experiment in the actual space of a given problem, or a realistic simulation of the problem environment. Therefore, it must have knowledge of the problem environment (or simulator) during the learning process. This information is given to the agent, through what is called *state* in the reinforcement learning nomenclature. In other words, a state is a variable that communicates characteristic information about the problem environment to the agent.

But, how does the agent learn as it interacts with the problem environment? The same way humans do when we are thrown into a new environment, one in which we have no theory or principles to stand on: by repeated trial-and-error interactions.

For example in the case of an autopilot system, we would train a reinforcement learning agent by giving it control of an airplane in a simulated environment. We would then run many simulations of the airplane traveling in various conditions, in each simulation giving the agent full control over steering the airplane. At first, the agent makes random steering actions, likely crashing the plane and ending the simulation. After many rounds of this type, the agent slowly starts learning how to steer correctly to achieve the goal of reaching a predefined destination point. In essence, in navigating the problem environment in pursuit of the desired goal, the reinforcement learning agent takes a sequence of *actions* in a trial-and-error fashion.

Of crucial importance here is the fact that it is the entire sequence of actions taken together that we want to lead successfully to accomplishing the goal. In the case of the autopilot system for example, the agent might take tens of thousands of actions before an eventual crash. And, as you might imagine, it is not at all trivial to identify which individual action or group of actions were responsible for the crash.

This brings us to an important question: how can we communicate an abstract goal (e.g., "reach destination safely") to the agent, so it can learn through many simulations the correct sorts of actions to take? In the reinforcement learning framework, we translate the desired goal into a series of numerical values called *rewards*. These reward values provide feedback to the agent at each step of a simulation run. Essentially, they tell the agent how well it is accomplishing the desired goal, helping the agent eventually learn the correct sequence of actions necessary to achieve it. In other words, a reward is a numerical value given to the reinforcement learning agent after it takes an action, to communicate to the agent whether we think the taken action has helped or hindered its accomplishment of the desired goal.

Note that it is completely up to us (humans) to decide on the reward structure. Intuitively, we want a reward for a given action to be larger for those actions that get us closer to accomplishing our goal (and less for those actions that do not). Designing a good reward structure is therefore crucial in solving any reinforcement learning problem as this is the (only) way we communicate our desired goal to the agent.

States, actions, and rewards are three fundamentals concepts in reinforcement learning that connect together to create a feedback system that, when properly engineered, allows us to train an agent to accomplish a task. The agent, based on the feedback it receives during training via our designed reward structure, learns how to take reward-maximizing actions that eventually lead to the desired goal. To further conceptualize these fundamental ideas, in what follows, we give several examples using the reinforcement learning applications introduced in Sect. "Reinforcement Learning Applications".

States, Actions, and Rewards in Gridworld

For any given Gridworld as shown in Figs. 8.1 and 8.2, knowledge of the agent's current location is enough to fully describe the problem environment. Hence, a state in this case consists of the horizontal and vertical coordinates of the black circle on the map. Recall that the robot in Gridworld is only allowed to move one unit up, down, left or right. These define the set of actions that the Gridworld agent can take. Note that depending on the agent's location (state), only a subset of actions may be available to the agent. For instance, if the agent is at the top-left corner of the map, it will only be allowed to go one unit right or down.

We can design a variety of reward structures to communicate our goal to the agent, that is, to reach the target (green square) in an efficient manner while avoiding the hazards (red squares). For example, we can assign a relatively-small-in-magnitude negative value (e.g., -1) to all actions (one unit movement) that lead to a non-goal *and* non-hazard state, a larger-in-magnitude negative value (e.g., -100) for those actions leading to a hazard state, and a non-negative number (e.g., 0) to actions leading to the goal state itself. This way, the agent is incentivized not to step on hazard squares (as its reward will be reduced by 100 each time it does so), and to reach the goal state in as few steps as possible (since walking over each white square still reduces its reward by 1).

To summarize, beginning at a state (location) in Gridworld, an action is taken to move the agent to a new state. For taking this action and moving to the new state, the agent receives a reward.

States, Actions, and Rewards in Cart–Pole

In the cart–pole problem described in Sect. "Automatic Control", a state is a complete set of information about the cart and pole's position. This includes the cart position, the cart velocity, the angle of the pole measured as its deviation from the vertical position, and the angular velocity of the pole. While these are technically continuous values, in practice they are finely discretized. It is important to note that in order to solve the cart–pole problem in a reinforcement learning framework, we need not make any assumptions about the environment, e.g., the fact that gravity exists, its precise force, etc.

The range of actions in the cart–pole example is completely defined by the available range of motions of the machine being directly controlled. In the example shown in the left panel of Fig. 8.3, the agent can keep the cart still, or move it one unit to the left or right along the horizontal axis. One common choice of reward structure in this case is as follows: at every state at which the angle between the pole and the horizontal axis is above a certain threshold, the agent is rewarded 1 point, and 0 otherwise. Therefore, beginning at a state (a specific configuration of the four system descriptors mentioned above), an action is taken (the cart is kept still or moved), and a new state of the system arises. For taking this action and moving to the new state, the agent receives a reward.

States, Actions, and Rewards in Chess

In playing the game of Chess, a state is any (legal) configuration of all (remaining) white and black pieces on the board, and an action is a legal move of any of current pieces on the board according to the rules of Chess. In this case, one reward structure to induce our agent to learn how to win could be as follows: any move made that does not immediately lead to the goal state (checkmating the opponent) receives a reward of -1, while a move that successfully checkmates the opponent receives a large positive reward (e.g., 10,000).

States, Actions, and Rewards in Radiotherapy Planning

In radiation therapy (discussed in Sect. "Automated Planning of Radiation Treatment"), a state consists of all information regarding the exact size and location of the tumor, as well as the existence of any structural damage to the surrounding healthy tissues. The state information is typically captured prior to each radiotherapy session using radiological imaging modalities such as CT-scans or MRIs. The reinforcement learning agent will then take an action in the form of irradiating the tumor at a specific angle/dose. A possible reward structure could be as follows: the agent receives a positive reward (e.g., $+2$) for every unit reduction in the volume of the tumor, and a smaller (in magnitude) negative reward (e.g., -1) for every unit increase in the volume of healthy tissue damaged as a result of radiation.

Mathematical Notation

Having discussed the fundamental concepts of reinforcement learning (states, actions, and rewards) in the previous section, we are now ready to introduce notation that will allow us to represent each of these concepts algebraically. For simplicity, we assume (for the time being) that any given reinforcement learning problem only has a finite number of states and actions. We will denote the set of all states by

$$\mathcal{S} = \{\sigma_1, \sigma_2, \ldots, \sigma_n\} \tag{8.1}$$

and the set of all actions by

$$\mathcal{A} = \{\alpha_1, \alpha_2, \ldots, \alpha_m\}. \tag{8.2}$$

At the kth step in solving a reinforcement learning problem, the agent begins at a state $s_k \in \mathcal{S}$ and takes an action $a_k \in \mathcal{A}$ that moves the system to a state $s_{k+1} \in \mathcal{S}$. It is important not to confuse the s notation with the σ notation in (8.1), and the a notation with the α notation in (8.2). The notation s_k is a variable denoting the state at which the kth step of the procedure begins and thus can be any of the possible realized states in $\mathcal{S} = \{\sigma_1, \sigma_2, \ldots, \sigma_n\}$. Similarly, the notation a_k is a variable denoting the action taken at the kth step, which is one of the permissible actions from the set $\mathcal{A} = \{\alpha_1, \alpha_2, \ldots, \alpha_m\}$.

Recall that the mechanism by which an agent learns the best action to take in a given state is the reward structure. We use the notation r_k to denote the reward an agent receives at the kth step. In general, r_k is a function of the initial state at the kth step of the process as well as the action taken by the reinforcement learning agent at this step

$$r_k = f(s_k, a_k). \tag{8.3}$$

In solving a reinforcement learning problem, an agent goes through a sequence of events at each step. In the beginning, the agent starts at an initial state s_1 and takes an action denoted by a_1 that changes the state of the problem to s_2. For taking the action a_1 at state s_1, the agent also receives the reward r_1. At the next (i.e., second) step, the agent starts at state s_2, takes the action a_2, receives the reward r_2, and moves to s_3. This sequential process is summarized visually in Fig. 8.7. Taken together a sequence of such steps, ending either when a goal state is reached (as in Gridworld or Chess) or after a maximum number of iterations is completed (as in the cart–pole example) is referred to in the language of reinforcement learning as an *episode*.

It must be noted that not all reinforcement learning problems are *deterministic* in nature, where one realized action a_k at a given state s_k always leads to the same next state s_{k+1}. In *stochastic* reinforcement learning problems, a given action at a state may lead to different conclusions. For example, a robot may perform a given action (e.g., accelerate forward one unit of thrust) at a state and reach different outcomes due to things such as inconsistencies in the application of this action,

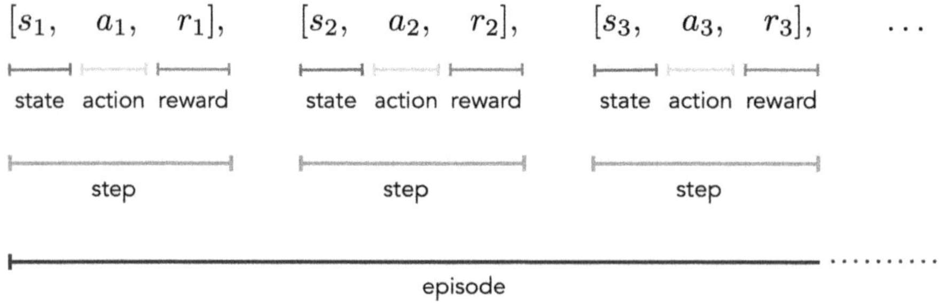

Fig. 8.7 An illustrative summary of the reinforcement learning nomenclature and notation introduced thus far

sensor issues, friction, etc. Almost the same modeling discussed in the section captures this variability for such stochastic problems, with the main difference being that the reward function must also necessarily be a function of the state s_{k+1} in addition to s_k and a_k, i.e.,

$$r_k = f\left(s_k, a_k, s_{k+1}\right). \tag{8.4}$$

Bellman's Equation

With notation out of the way, we are now ready to address perhaps the most important question in reinforcement learning: how do we actually train the agent? The answer is—like any other machine learning problem—through optimizing an appropriate cost function. However, unlike other machine learning problems such as linear or logistic regression, here we cannot directly work out an exact parameterized form of the cost function. Instead, we formalize a certain attribute that we want this function to ideally have and, working backward, we can arrive at a method for computing it.

Let us define $Q(s_1, a_1)$ as the maximum total reward possible if we begin at the state s_1 and take the action a_1. Recall that taking the action a_1 brings us to some state s_2, and the agent receives some reward r_1. Therefore, $Q(s_1, a_1)$ can be calculated as the sum of the realized reward r_1 plus the largest possible total reward from all the proceeding steps starting from the state s_2. Invoking the definition of the Q function, this latter quantity can be written as

$$\max_{i \in \Omega(s_2)} Q\left(s_2, \alpha_i\right), \tag{8.5}$$

where $\Omega(s_2)$ denotes the index set for all valid actions that can be taken when the agent is at the state s_2. Writing out the equality above algebraically, we then have

$$Q(s_1, a_1) = r_1 + \max_{i \in \Omega(s_2)} Q\left(s_2, \alpha_i\right). \tag{8.6}$$

Note that the expression in (8.6) holds generally regardless of what state and action we begin with. In other words, at the kth step of the process, we can write

$$Q(s_k, a_k) = r_k + \max_{i \in \Omega(s_{k+1})} Q\left(s_{k+1}, \alpha_i\right). \tag{8.7}$$

This recursive definition of the Q function is typically referred to as Bellman's equation. At first glance, this recursive equation seems to aid little in helping us determine the optimal Q function since Q appears on both sides of (8.7). Luckily, we can leverage the agent's intrinsic ability to interact with the problem environment to resolve Q. The idea is to initialize Q to some (random) value, run a large number of episodes, and update Q via Bellman's recursive equation as we go along. This essentially constitutes the training phase of reinforcement learning. In the next section, we discuss, in full detail, how to resolve the Q function—or in other words, train the RL agent—via the so-called Q-learning algorithm.

The Basic Q-Learning Algorithm

When dealing with reinforcement learning problems with a finite number of states and actions, the Q function can be represented as a two-dimensional matrix. Recall from (8.1) and (8.2) that we denote the set of all states as $\mathcal{S} = \{\sigma_1, \sigma_2, \ldots, \sigma_n\}$, and the set of all possible actions as $\mathcal{A} = \{\alpha_1, \alpha_2, \ldots, \alpha_m\}$. Therefore, Q can be represented as the $n \times m$ matrix

$$\begin{bmatrix} Q(\sigma_1, \alpha_1) & Q(\sigma_1, \alpha_2) & \cdots & Q(\sigma_1, \alpha_m) \\ Q(\sigma_2, \alpha_1) & Q(\sigma_2, \alpha_2) & \cdots & Q(\sigma_2, \alpha_m) \\ \vdots & \vdots & \ddots & \vdots \\ Q(\sigma_n, \alpha_1) & Q(\sigma_n, \alpha_2) & \cdots & Q(\sigma_n, \alpha_m) \end{bmatrix}, \tag{8.8}$$

which is indexed by all possible actions along its columns, and all possible states along its rows. In the beginning, this matrix can be initialized at random (or at zero). Next, by running through an episode of simulation

$$[s_1,\ a_1,\ r_1], \quad [s_2,\ a_2,\ r_2], \quad [s_3,\ a_3,\ r_3], \quad \ldots, \tag{8.9}$$

we generate data that can be used to resolve the optimal Q function step-by-step via the recursive definition in (8.7). With the matrix Q initialized, the agent takes its first action *at random* for which it receives the reward r_1. Based on this reward, we can update $Q(s_1, a_1)$ via (8.6), as

$$Q(s_1, a_1) \leftarrow r_1 + \max_{i \in \Omega(s_2)} Q(s_2,\ \alpha_i). \tag{8.10}$$

The agent then takes its second action (once again at random) for which it receives the reward r_2, and we update $Q(s_2, a_2)$ via

$$Q(s_2, a_2) \leftarrow r_2 + \max_{i \in \Omega(s_3)} Q(s_3,\ \alpha_i). \tag{8.11}$$

This sequential update process continues until a goal state is reached or a maximum number of steps are taken. When the current episode ends, we begin a new episode and continue updating Q.

After performing enough training episodes, our Q matrix/function eventually becomes optimal, since (by construction) it will satisfy the desired recursive definition for all state–action pairs. Notice, in order for Q to be optimal for all state–action pairs, every such pair must be visited at least once. In practice, one must typically cycle through each pair multiple times in order for Q to be trained appropriately or employ function approximators to generalize from a small subset of state–action pairs to the entire space.

In summary, by running through a large number of episodes (and so through as many state–action pairs as many times as possible), and updating Q at each step using the recursive Bellman's equation, we learn Q by trial-and-error interactions with the environment. How well our computations converge to the true Q function relies heavily on how well we sample the state–action spaces through our trial-and-error interactions. The pseudocode for the basic version of the Q-learning algorithm is given below.

The basic Q-learning algorithm

```
 1: Initialize Q
 2: Set the number of episodes E
 3: Set the maximum number of steps per episodes T
 4: for e = 1, 2, ..., E do
 5:     k = 1
 6:     Select a random initial state s_1
 7:     while goal state not reached and k ≤ T do
 8:         Select an action a_k from Ω(s_k) at random
 9:         Record the resulting state s_{k+1} and corresponding reward r_k
10:         Q(s_k, a_k) ← r_k + max_{i∈Ω(s_{k+1})} Q(s_{k+1}, α_i)
11:         k ← k + 1
12:     end while
13: end for
```

Example 8.1 (Applying Q-Learning to Gridworld) In this example, we use Q-learning to train an agent for the small Gridworld map shown in the left panel of Fig. 8.2. Recall that with Gridworld, our goal is to train the agent (shown in black) to efficiently reach the goal square (shown in green) while avoiding the hazard squares (shown in red), starting from any square on the grid. Here, each state can be represented by the coordinates of the agent's location on the map as shown in the left panel of Fig. 8.8. The total number of states, therefore, equals the number of squares on the grid, i.e., $n = 25$. As shown in the right panel of Fig. 8.8, the agent can take one of four actions: move up, down, left, and right one square at a time. Hence, $m = 4$.

Next, we initialize a 25×4 matrix Q with all zero entries and set the number of training episodes E and the number of steps per episode T both to 100. We will discuss briefly how to tune these parameters in

(continued)

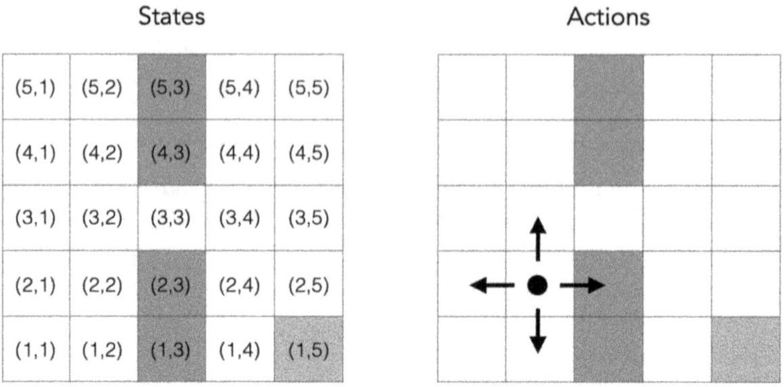

Fig. 8.8 All the possible states (left panel) and actions (right panel) for the Gridworld shown originally in the left panel of Fig. 8.2

Example 8.1 (continued)
Sect. "Tuning the Q-Learning Parameters". Finally, we preset reward values for the agent at each location on the grid as

$$r_k = \begin{cases} -0.001 & \text{if on standard square,} \\ -1 & \text{if on hazard square,} \\ 0 & \text{if at goal} \end{cases} \tag{8.12}$$

and run the Q-learning algorithm. The initial and final Q matrices (at the beginning of episode 1 and at the end of episode 100) are displayed in Table 8.1.

The Testing Phase of Q-Learning

In Example 8.1, we saw how to train a reinforcement learning agent via Q-learning. In this section, we study how the agent should leverage the learned Q matrix/function to navigate the problem environment.

Recall from our discussion in Sect. "Bellman's Equation" that $Q(s_k, a_k)$ is the maximum total reward possible if the agent begins at s_k and takes the action a_k. Therefore, to maximize the overall reward, we should choose the action a_k such that $Q(s_k, a_k)$ has the largest possible value, or equivalently

$$a_k = \alpha_{i^\star}, \tag{8.13}$$

Table 8.1 The initial (left) and final (right) Q matrices associated with Example 8.1. Here, each row is a state and each column an action. The Q matrix on the left was initialized at zero. The Q matrix on the right was resolved after running 100 episodes of the Q-learning algorithm

	Down $\downarrow$	Up $\uparrow$	Left $\leftarrow$	Right $\rightarrow$	Down $\downarrow$	Up $\uparrow$	Left $\leftarrow$	Right $\rightarrow$
(1, 1)	0	0	0	0	−0.008	−0.007	−0.008	−0.007
(1, 2)	0	0	0	0	−0.007	−0.006	−0.008	−1.001
(1, 3)	0	0	0	0	−1.001	−1.002	−0.007	−0.001
(1, 4)	0	0	0	0	−0.001	−0.002	−1.001	0
(1, 5)	0	0	0	0	0	0	0	0
(2, 1)	0	0	0	0	−0.008	−0.006	−0.007	−0.006
(2, 2)	0	0	0	0	−0.007	−0.005	−0.007	−1.002
(2, 3)	0	0	0	0	−1.001	−0.004	−0.006	−0.002
(2, 4)	0	0	0	0	−0.001	−0.003	−1.002	−0.001
(2, 5)	0	0	0	0	0	−0.002	−0.002	−0.001
(3, 1)	0	0	0	0	−0.007	−0.007	−0.006	−0.005
(3, 2)	0	0	0	0	−0.006	−0.006	−0.006	−0.004
(3, 3)	0	0	0	0	−1.002	−1.004	−0.005	−0.003
(3, 4)	0	0	0	0	−0.002	−0.004	−0.004	−0.002
(3, 5)	0	0	0	0	−0.001	−0.003	−0.003	−0.002
(4, 1)	0	0	0	0	−0.006	−0.008	−0.007	−0.006
(4, 2)	0	0	0	0	−0.005	−0.007	−0.007	−1.004
(4, 3)	0	0	0	0	−0.004	−1.005	−0.006	−0.004
(4, 4)	0	0	0	0	−0.003	−0.005	−1.004	−0.003
(4, 5)	0	0	0	0	−0.002	−0.004	−0.004	−0.003
(5, 1)	0	0	0	0	−0.007	−0.008	−0.008	−0.007
(5, 2)	0	0	0	0	−0.006	−0.007	−0.008	−1.005
(5, 3)	0	0	0	0	−1.004	−1.005	−0.007	−0.005
(5, 4)	0	0	0	0	−0.004	−0.005	−1.005	−0.004
(5, 5)	0	0	0	0	−0.003	−0.004	−0.005	−0.004

where

$$i^{\star} = \underset{i \in \Omega(s_k)}{\operatorname{argmax}} \; Q\left(s_k, \alpha_i\right). \tag{8.14}$$

Equations (8.13) and (8.14) define a *policy* for the reinforcement learning agent to utilize when it finds itself at any state s_k. Once Q is resolved properly and sufficiently, the agent can use this policy to take actions that allow it to travel in a reward-maximizing path of states until it reaches the goal (or a maximum number of steps are taken).

Example 8.2 (Testing the Reinforcement Learning Agent in Gridworld) In this example, we use the Q matrix learned in Example 8.1 and shown on the right side of Table 8.1 in order to test how the reinforcement learning agent navigates the Gridworld, starting at any given location (state) on the board. Here, we initialize the agent at $s_1 = (2, 2)$.

As shown in Fig. 8.9, by inspecting the row associated with s_1 in the Q matrix, we can easily see that the entry in the " Up/↑ " column has the largest value in the entire row (i.e., −0.005). Therefore, the optimal action to take at this state is to move the agent up one unit, to $s_2 = (3, 2)$. Next, we examine the row associated with $s_2 = (3, 2)$. Now the largest entry is −0.004, which lies in the " Right/→ " column, meaning that the best action to take is move the agent one unit to the right to a new state $s_3 = (3, 3)$. Once again, the entry under the " Right/→" column is the largest in the row associated with s_3, and the agent continues to move right to $s_4 = (3, 4)$.

As shown in Fig. 8.10, along the row associated with s_4, the two actions of moving " Down/↓ " or " Right/→ "share the same largest value of −0.002. In such circumstances, the agent can take either action, arriving at $s_4 = (2, 4)$ in the former case (shown in solid blue) or $s_4 = (3, 5)$ in the latter case (shown in dashed blue). This process is repeated until the target state is reached (or a pre-determined maximum number of steps are taken). Figure 8.11 shows all the possible paths the agent can take starting at $s_1 = (2, 2)$, all ending at the target state $s_7 = (1, 5)$.

	Down ↓	Up ↑	Left ←	Right →
(1, 1)	−0.008	−0.007	−0.008	−0.007
(1, 2)	−0.007	−0.006	−0.008	−1.001
(1, 3)	−1.001	−1.002	−0.007	−0.001
(1, 4)	−0.001	−0.002	−1.001	0
(1, 5)	0	0	0	0
(2, 1)	−0.008	−0.006	−0.007	−0.006
(2, 2)	−0.007	−0.005	−0.007	−1.002
(2, 3)	−1.001	−0.004	−0.006	−0.002
(2, 4)	−0.001	−0.003	−1.002	−0.001
(2, 5)	0	−0.002	−0.002	−0.001
(3, 1)	−0.007	−0.007	−0.006	−0.005
(3, 2)	−0.006	−0.006	−0.006	−0.004
(3, 3)	−1.002	−1.004	−0.005	−0.003
(3, 4)	−0.002	−0.004	−0.004	−0.002
(3, 5)	−0.001	−0.003	−0.003	−0.002
(4, 1)	−0.006	−0.008	−0.007	−0.006
[illegible]	[illegible]	−0.007	−0.007	[illegible]

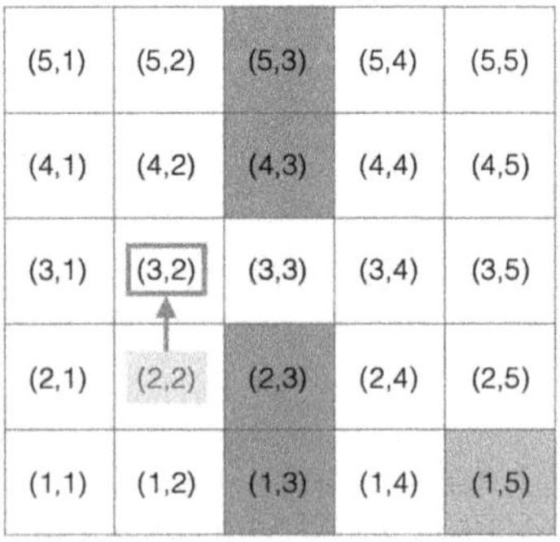

Fig. 8.9 Starting at state $s_1 = (2, 2)$, the agent looks up Q in search of the largest value along the row associated with s_1. In this case, −0.005 is the largest value that happens to fall under the " Up/↑ " column. Taking this recommended action, will take the agent to $s_2 = (3, 2)$

	Down ↓	Up ↑	Left ←	Right →
(1, 1)	−0.008	−0.007	−0.008	−0.007
(1, 2)	−0.007	−0.006	−0.008	−1.001
(1, 3)	−1.001	−1.002	−0.007	−0.001
(1, 4)	−0.001	−0.002	−1.001	0
(1, 5)	0	0	0	0
(2, 1)	−0.008	−0.006	−0.007	−0.006
(2, 2)	−0.007	−0.005	−0.007	−1.002
(2, 3)	−1.001	−0.004	−0.006	−0.002
(2, 4)	−0.001	−0.003	−1.002	−0.001
(2, 5)	0	−0.002	−0.002	−0.001
(3, 1)	−0.007	−0.007	−0.006	−0.005
(3, 2)	−0.006	−0.006	−0.006	−0.004
(3, 3)	−1.002	−1.004	−0.005	−0.003
(3, 4)	−0.002	−0.004	−0.004	−0.002
(3, 5)	−0.001	−0.003	−0.003	−0.002
(4, 1)	−0.006	−0.008	−0.007	−0.006
[illegible]	[illegible]	−0.007	−0.007	[illegible]

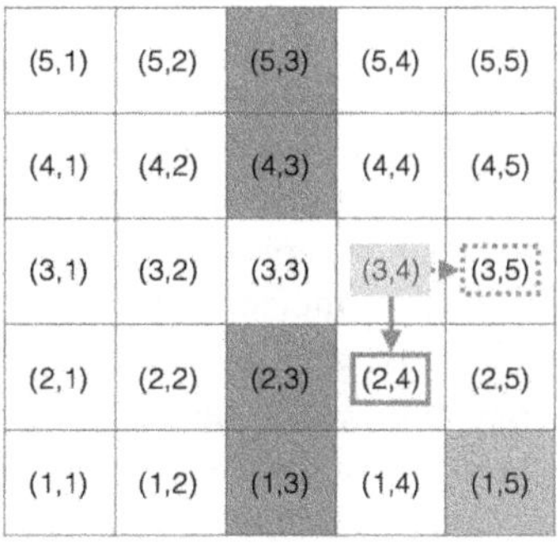

Fig. 8.10 The largest value along a given row in Q is not always unique. In such cases, the agent can choose any of the available optimal actions at random. Here, starting at (3, 4), the agent can move either down to (2, 4) or right to (3, 5)

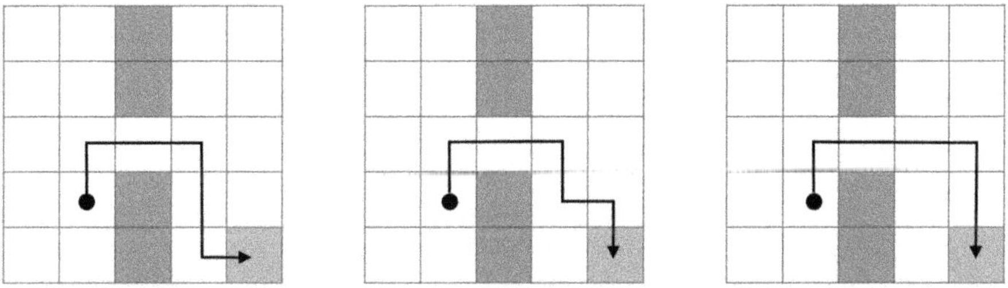

Fig. 8.11 Starting at $s_1 = (2, 2)$ and following the policy defined in (8.13) and (8.14), the agent has three paths to the target state shown in green

Tuning the Q-Learning Parameters

The basic Q-learning algorithm has a number of parameters to set. These include the number of maximum steps per episode of training T, as well as the total number of training episodes E. Each of these parameters can heavily influence the performance of the trained agent. On one end of the spectrum, if T is not set high enough, the agent may never reach the goal state. With a problem like Gridworld—where there is only one such state—this would be disastrous as the system (and Q) would never learn how to reach the goal. On the other hand, the training can take an extremely long time if the number of steps is set too large.

A similar story can be said for the number of episodes E: too small, and Q will not be learned properly, and too large results in much wasted time and computation.

As we will see later in the chapter, other variants of the basic Q-learning algorithm have additional parameters that need to be set as well.

To tune the Q-learning parameters, we need a *validation* strategy to evaluate the performance of our trained agent with different parameter settings. This validation strategy includes running a set of validation episodes, where each episode begins at a different starting position, and the agent transitions using the optimal policy. Calculating the average reward on a set of validation episodes at the completion of each training episode can then help us evaluate how a particular parameter setting affects the efficiency and speed of training.

Because a problem like the Gridworld discussed in Examples 8.1 and 8.2 has a small number of states, the number of steps T and episodes E can be kept relatively low. Ideally, however, we set both to a large number—as large as possible—given time and computational constraints.

Q-Learning Enhancements

In the previous section, we introduced the basic Q-learning algorithm as a means to approximate the fundamental Q function associated to every reinforcement learning problem. In this section, we continue our discussion and introduce two simple yet powerful enhancements to the basic Q-learning algorithm.

Recall that at the heart of the basic Q-learning algorithm is the following recursive update equation:

$$Q(s_k, a_k) = r_k + \max_{i \in \Omega(s_{k+1})} Q\left(s_{k+1}, \alpha_i\right), \tag{8.15}$$

where the term on the left hand side, i.e., $Q(s_k, a_k)$, stands for the maximum possible reward the agent receives if it starts at state s_k and takes action a_k. This is equal to the sum of the two terms on the right hand side of the equation: the first (r_k) stands for the immediate *short-term* reward the agent receives for taking action a_k at state s_k, and the second term stands for the maximum *long-term* reward the agent can potentially receive starting from state s_{k+1}.

Note that the recursive equation in (8.15) was originally derived assuming Q was optimal. This is clearly not true at first when we begin training[1] since we do not have knowledge of the optimal Q (that is why we have to train in the first place). Therefore, neither term on the left and right hand sides of (8.15) involving Q gives us a maximal value initially in the process. However, we can make several adjustments to the basic Q-learning algorithm to compensate for the fact that the optimal Q—and hence the validity of the recursive update equation—takes several episodes of simulation to resolve properly.

[1] Recall that Q is initialized randomly or at zero.

The Exploration–Exploitation Trade-Off

One glaring inefficiency in the basic Q-learning algorithm is the fact that the agent takes *random* actions during training (see line 8 of the basic Q-learning algorithm in Sect. "The Basic Q-Learning Algorithm"). This inefficiency becomes more palpable if we simply look at the total rewards per episode of training. In Fig. 8.12, we plot the total reward gained per episode of training for the small Gridworld in the left panel of Fig. 8.2. The rapid fluctuation in total reward per episode seen in this plot is a direct consequence of using random action selection for training the reinforcement learning agent. The average reward over time does not improve even though Q is getting more accurate as training proceeds. Adjacently, this means that the average amount of computation time stays roughly the same no matter how well we have resolved Q.

While training with random action selection does force the agent to explore the problem environment well during training, we never exploit the resolving Q matrix/function during training in order to take actions. It seems intuitive that after a while the agent does not need to rely completely on random action-taking. Instead, it can use the (partially) resolved Q to take proper actions while training. As Q becomes more and more close to optimal, this would clearly lower training time in later episodes, since the agent is now taking actions informed by the Q function/matrix instead of merely random ones.

The important question is: when should the agent start exploiting Q during training? We already have a sense of what happens if the agent never does this: training will be highly inefficient. On the other hand, if the agent starts exploiting Q *too soon* and *too much*, it might not explore enough of the state space of the problem to create a robust learner as the learning of Q would be heavily biased in favor of early successful episodes.

In practice, there are various ways of applying this exploration–exploitation trade-off for choosing actions during training. Most of these schemes use a simple

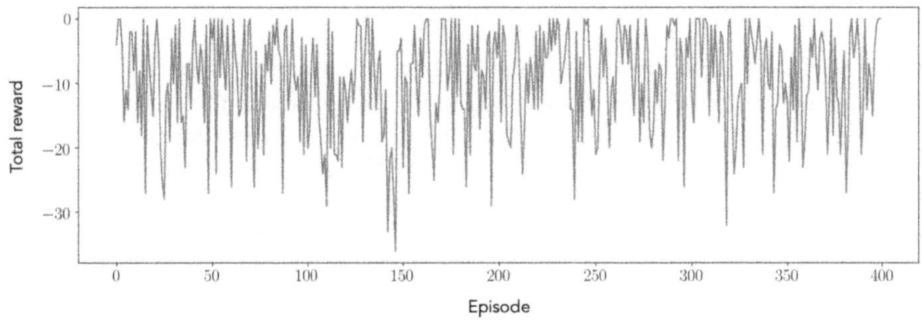

Fig. 8.12 The total reward per episode recorded during simulation after running the basic Q-learning algorithm for 400 episodes on the Gridworld shown originally in the left panel of Fig. 8.2

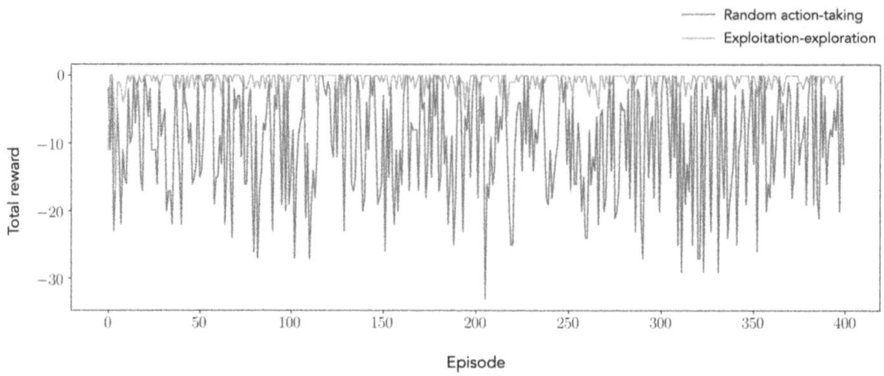

Fig. 8.13 Comparison of the random action-taking and exploitation–exploration modes of Q-learning. In this instance, the Q-learning algorithm using exploitation–exploration (in orange) completed 5 times faster than the basic version with strictly random action-taking (in blue)

stochastic switch: at each step of an episode of simulation, choose the next action randomly with a certain probability p, or via the optimal policy with probability $1 - p$. In the most naive approach, the probability p can be kept fixed at some value between 0 and 1 and used for all steps/episodes of training. More thoughtful implementations push p gradually toward zero as training proceeds, since the approximation of Q gets more reliable over time.

To see how much exploitation of Q helps make training more efficient, we repeat the process used to create Fig. 8.12, this time setting the exploration–exploitation probability p to 0.5 for all steps/episodes. As can be seen in Fig. 8.13, the exploration–exploitation method produces episodes with much greater stability (i.e., less fluctuation) and with far greater total reward.

The Short-Term Long-Term Reward Trade-Off

If it is true—at least in the first training episodes of Q-learning—that the long-term reward is not too reliable, then we can dampen its contribution to the update. This can be done by adding a parameter to the long-term reward, sometimes referred to as a penalty parameter or regularization parameter. This short-term long-term trade-off parameter is tacked on to the long-term reward and is often denoted by γ. With this trade-off parameter included, our recursion update formula now takes the following form:

$$Q(s_k, a_k) = r_k + \gamma \cdot \max_{i \in \Omega(s_{k+1})} Q\left(s_{k+1}, \alpha_i\right). \tag{8.16}$$

We constrain γ to lie between 0 and 1, so that by scaling it up and down, we can tune the influence that short-term and long-term rewards have on how Q is learned. In particular, by setting γ to a smaller value, we assign more weight to the contribution of the short-term reward r_k. In this case, the agent learns to take a more *greedy* approach to accomplishing the goal, at each state taking the next step that essentially maximizes the short-term reward only.

On the other hand, by setting γ close to 1, we essentially have our original update formula back, where we take into account equal contributions of both short-term and long-term rewards. As with the exploration–exploitation trade-off, one can either set γ to a fixed value for all steps/episodes during training or change its value from episode to episode according to a predefined schedule. Sometimes setting γ to some value smaller than 1 helps proving mathematical convergence of Q-learning. In practice, however, γ is usually set close to 1 (if not 1), and we just tinker with the exploration–exploitation probability because in the end both trade-offs (exploration–exploitation and short-term long-term reward) address the same issue: our initial distrust of Q. Integrating both trade-off modifications into the basic Q-learning algorithm, we have the following enhanced version of Q-learning given in the pseudocode below.

The enhanced Q-learning algorithm

```
Initialize Q
Set the number of episodes E
Set the maximum number of steps per episodes T
Set the exploration-exploitation probability p ∈ [0, 1]
Set the short-term long-term reward trade-off γ ∈ [0, 1]
for e = 1, 2, ..., E do
    k = 1
    Select a random initial state s_1
    while goal state not reached and k ≤ T do
        choose a random number r ∈ [0, 1]
        if r ≤ p then
            Select an action a_k from Ω(s_k) at random
        else
            Select the action a_k that maximizes Q(s_k, a_k)
        end if
        Record the resulting state s_{k+1} and corresponding reward r_k
        Q(s_k, a_k) ← r_k + γ · max_{i∈Ω(s_{k+1})} Q(s_{k+1}, α_i)
        k ← k + 1
    end while
end for
```

Tackling Problems with Large State Spaces

In the previous section, we introduced two enhancements that make Q-learning more efficient. However, in many reinforcement learning scenarios, the state space of the problem is so large that these enhancements alone cannot make Q-learning tractable. Take the game of Chess, for instance, where each state is a configuration of the pieces on the board. It is estimated[2] that the number of such configurations is of the general order of $\frac{64!}{32!(8!)^2(2!)^6}$, or roughly 10^{43}. Storing and computing with such a large matrix Q is extremely challenging, if not *practically* impossible. To make matters worse, sometimes reinforcement learning problems have continuous state spaces, which makes representing Q as a matrix *theoretically* impossible (since such a matrix would need to have infinitely many rows). In this section, we discuss the crucial role supervised learning plays in ameliorating this issue, allowing us to extend the reinforcement learning paradigm to problems with very large state spaces.

To cast the problem formally, suppose we have an $n \times m$ matrix Q as shown originally in (8.8), where n is prohibitively large (or potentially infinite). One common way to address this problem is to use supervised learning in order to learn m compact algebraic expressions, one for each column in Q. Using this strategy, the jth column of Q

$$\begin{bmatrix} Q\left(\sigma_1, \alpha_j\right) \\ Q\left(\sigma_2, \alpha_j\right) \\ \vdots \\ Q\left(\sigma_n, \alpha_j\right) \end{bmatrix} \tag{8.17}$$

will be replaced by a single mathematical function $q_j(s)$ whose evaluation at $s = \sigma_i$ (approximately) equals $Q(\sigma_i, \alpha_j)$. In other words, the (i, j)th entry in Q that was previously represented by $Q(\sigma_i, \alpha_j)$ is now represented by $q_j(\sigma_i)$ where $q_j(\cdot)$ is a mathematical function (e.g., $q_j(s) = 1 - 2s$). Note that the input of the function $q_j(s)$ can take on *any* values from a finite set (e.g., $\mathcal{S} = \{\sigma_1, \sigma_2, \ldots, \sigma_n\}$) or even an infinite range. If the algebraic equation of $q_j(s)$ is known, the agent can simply plug any state value into the function and read the output, as opposed to having to look it up in a very large matrix.

The question then becomes: how can we learn the equations of $q_1(s)$, $q_2(s)$, ..., $q_m(s)$? In the simplest case, we can assume that all these functions can be modeled *linearly* and *independently* of each other. In other words, the jth function $q_j(s)$ can be modeled as

---

[2] The pioneering electrical engineer Claude Shannon, who is regarded as the father of information theory, published a seminal paper in 1950 entitled *Programming a Computer for Playing Chess* [2] in which he points out the intractability of the approach of defining a "dictionary" for all possible positions in Chess.

$$q_j(s) = w_{0,j} + w_{1,j}\, s, \tag{8.18}$$

where $w_{0,j}$ and $w_{1,j}$ are tunable weights or parameters. At each step of Q-learning, rather than updating some $Q(\sigma_k, \alpha_j)$, we update the parameters of the corresponding function $q_j(s)$—typically via online learning—such that

$$q_j(\sigma_k) \approx r_k + \max_{i \in \Omega(s_{k+1})} q_i\left(s_{k+1}\right). \tag{8.19}$$

Note that this is very similar to the linear regression setup described in Chap. 4 where the input–output pairs[3] associated with the linear function q_j arise occasionally in a sequential manner, as the agent navigates the problem environment.

Sometimes a linear function is not flexible enough to model $q_j(s)$ accurately. In such cases, we may choose nonlinear function approximators and rewrite (8.18) as

$$q_j(s) = f_j(s; \mathcal{W}_j), \tag{8.20}$$

where $f_j(s; \mathcal{W}_j)$ is a parameterized nonlinear function in s (e.g., a neural network) whose parameters are stored in the set $\mathcal{W}_j$. When using neural networks and depending on the reinforcement learning problem being solved, we have the choice of learning the f_j's independently (i.e., one network per action) or jointly (i.e., one network for all actions whose weights are shared across all state functions).

Problems

8.1 Define States, Actions, and Rewards

For each of the following, define: (i) the state space and (ii) the action space of the problem, as well as (iii) a proper reward structure for the reinforcement learning agent to achieve its goal. See Sect. "States, Actions, and Rewards in Radiotherapy Planning" for an example.

(a) The lunar lander problem as described in Sect. "Automatic Control"
(b) Pattern-cutting in robotic surgery as described in Sect. "Autonomous Robotic Surgery"

8.2 *Q*-Learning in a New Gridworld

In Example 8.1, we learned the Q matrix associated with the Gridworld shown in Fig. 8.8. In this exercise, you will apply Q-learning to a new Gridworld map shown in Fig. 8.14. Specifically, you should:

[3] Here, the input is σ_k, and the output is $r_k + \max_{i \in \Omega(s_{k+1})} q_i\left(s_{k+1}\right)$.

Fig. 8.14 Figure associated with Exercise 8.2

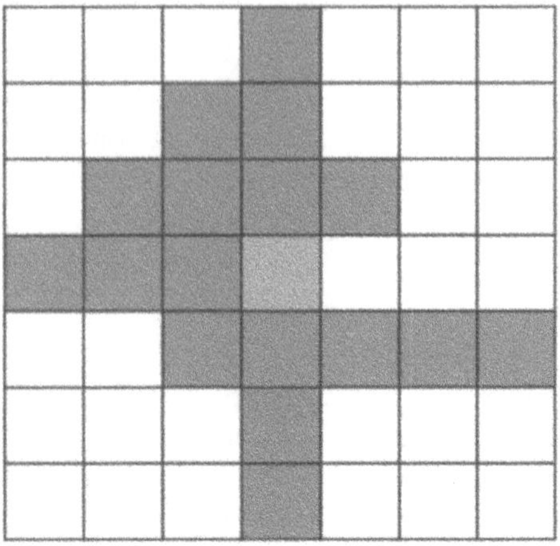

(a) Initialize the Q matrix at random and run the Q-learning algorithm to resolve Q
(b) Use the resolved Q to test the reinforcement learning agent placed initially at each of the four corners of the Gridworld. Does the agent navigate the map as expected? If not, why?

8.3 Q-Learning Enhancements
In Sects. "The Exploration–Exploitation Trade-Off" and "The Short-Term Long-Term Reward Trade-Off", we discussed two enhancements to improve the efficiency of the basic Q-learning algorithm, namely, the introduction of the exploitation–exploration probability p, and the short-term long-term reward trade-off parameter γ.

(a) Show that the enhanced Q-learning algorithm (whose pseudocode is shown in the end of Sect. "Q-Learning Enhancements") reduces to the basic Q-learning algorithm when both p and γ are set to 1.
(b) Describe what happens when both p and γ are set to 0.

8.4 Calculating the Size of Action Space in Chess
We saw in Sect. "Tackling Problems with Large State Spaces" that the *state* space of Chess is gargantuan, roughly in the order of 10^{43}. This motivated the use of function approximators in place of writing Q explicitly in matrix format. What about the *action* space of Chess? Is the action space, too, prohibitively large? In this exercise, you will answer this question by estimating (an upper bound on) the size of the action space in Chess using the information provided in Table 8.2 and noting that the Chess board itself is an 8×8 square.

Table 8.2 The number (per player) of pieces in Chess along with a description of how each piece is allowed to move on the board. This table is associated with Exercise 8.4

Name	Symbol	No. of pieces	Legal moves
Pawn	♙	8	1 square up; 2 squares up (first move only); 1 square forward diagonally when capturing an enemy piece (*en passant* capturing)
Rook	♖	2	Any number of squares horizontally or vertically; Castling with the King or the Queen
Knight	♘	2	2 squares vertically and 1 square horizontally; 2 squares horizontally and 1 square vertically
Bishop	♗	2	Any number of squares diagonally
Queen	♕	1	Any number of squares vertically, horizontally, or diagonally; Castling with a rook
King	♔	1	1 square vertically, horizontally, or diagonally; Castling with a rook

References

1. Murali A, Sen S, Kehoe B, et al. Learning by observation for surgical subtasks: multilateral cutting of 3D viscoelastic and 2D orthotropic tissue phantoms. In: Proceedings of the 2015 IEEE international conference on robotics and automation; 2015.p. 1202–9
2. Shannon CE. Programming a computer playing chess. Philos Mag. 1959;41(312)

Index

R. Borhani et al., *Fundamentals of Machine Learning and Deep Learning in Medicine*, https://doi.org/10.1007/978-3-031-19502-0

N

GPSR Compliance
The European Union's (EU) General Product Safety Regulation (GPSR) is a set of rules that requires consumer products to be safe and our obligations to ensure this.

If you have any concerns about our products, you can contact us on

ProductSafety@springernature.com

In case Publisher is established outside the EU, the EU authorized representative is:

Springer Nature Customer Service Center GmbH
Europaplatz 3
69115 Heidelberg, Germany

www.ingramcontent.com/pod-product-compliance
Ingram Content Group UK Ltd.
Pitfield, Milton Keynes, MK11 3LW, UK
UKHW020636051126
16351UKWH00010B/49
9783031195037